HOW TO STAY FIT AND HEALTHY DURING
Pregnancy

HOW TO STAY FIT AND HEALTHY DURING
Pregnancy

Kate Brian

Medical Adviser - Dr Sarah Jean Prince MRCOG
Fitness Adviser - Ellie Brown, Founder, Greenwich Fitness & Pilates

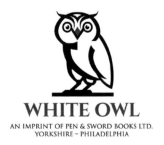

WHITE OWL
AN IMPRINT OF PEN & SWORD BOOKS LTD.
YORKSHIRE – PHILADELPHIA

First published in Great Britain in 2019 by
Pen and Sword WHITE OWL
An imprint of
Pen & Sword Books Ltd
Yorkshire - Philadelphia

Copyright © Kate Brian, 2019

ISBN 978 1 52673 209 5

Typeset in 11/14 pts Cormorant Infant
by Aura Technology and Software Services, India

Printed and bound in India by Replika Press Pvt. Ltd.

Pen & Sword Books Ltd incorporates the Imprints of Pen & Sword Books Archaeology, Atlas, Aviation, Battleground, Discovery, Family History, History, Maritime, Military, Naval, Politics, Railways, Select, Transport, True Crime, Fiction, Frontline Books, Leo Cooper, Praetorian Press, Seaforth Publishing, Wharncliffe and White Owl.

For a complete list of Pen & Sword titles please contact

PEN & SWORD BOOKS LIMITED
47 Church Street, Barnsley, South Yorkshire, S70 2AS, England
E-mail: enquiries@pen-and-sword.co.uk
Website: www.pen-and-sword.co.uk

or

PEN AND SWORD BOOKS
1950 Lawrence Rd, Havertown, PA 19083, USA
E-mail: Uspen-and-sword@casematepublishers.com
Website: www.penandswordbooks.com

Contents

CHAPTER ONE

Your Changing Body

Pregnancy is a huge, life-changing step and a time of physical and emotional change. From the moment a single sperm breaks through the outer surface of an egg to fertilize it, your body begins to adjust to your new status. Keeping fit and healthy when you are pregnant is important for both you and your baby, and helps to prepare your body for giving birth. Often women are uncertain about what they should and should not do in pregnancy, but being aware of the changes taking place in your body will help you to understand how to maintain your health and fitness. Although there may be some limitations on what you can do and what you feel like doing, most women are able to remain active in pregnancy. Whether you are a fitness addict who is worried that pregnancy may curb your exercise regime or someone whose idea of exercise is walking to the corner shop, whether you follow a clean eating regime or tend to grab whatever is available when you are hungry, you

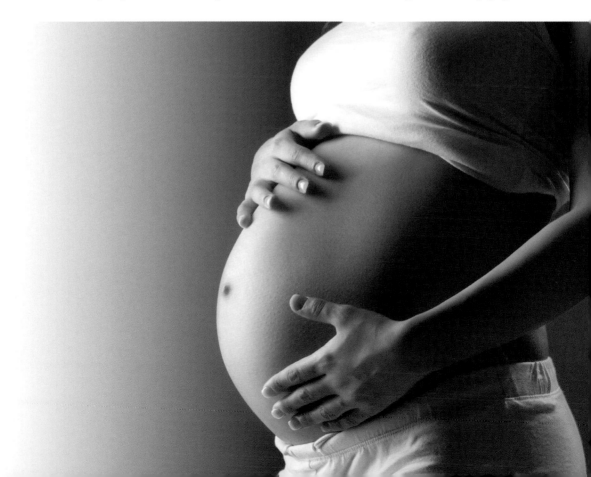

can benefit from following evidence-based advice about a healthy diet and an active lifestyle when you are expecting.

Your pregnancy will dominate the next nine months of your life. Lasting around forty weeks, pregnancy is divided into three separate periods known as trimesters, each of around three months. The first trimester covers the first three months of pregnancy, the second goes from four to six months and the third from seven to nine months. How active you can be and what type of exercise you may want to take is likely to change during these different phases of your pregnancy.

EARLY SIGNS OF PREGNANCY

For most women, the first sign that you are expecting a baby is a missed period. At this point, your pregnancy hormone levels are still rising and you may not experience any of the other signs of early pregnancy that you have heard about. It is possible that you may have some spotting or light bleeding in very early pregnancy when the fertilized egg implants into the womb lining and this is known as implantation bleeding. Women sometimes assume that they could not be pregnant if they bleed and you should always seek medical advice about bleeding, but it is not uncommon to have some spotting or light bleeding in the first few months of pregnancy.

If you think you could be pregnant, you can buy a home test at a local pharmacy or supermarket to check. Home tests are generally very reliable as long as the instructions are followed properly, but some are more sensitive than others and can pick up a pregnancy from a sample of urine sooner when hormone levels are

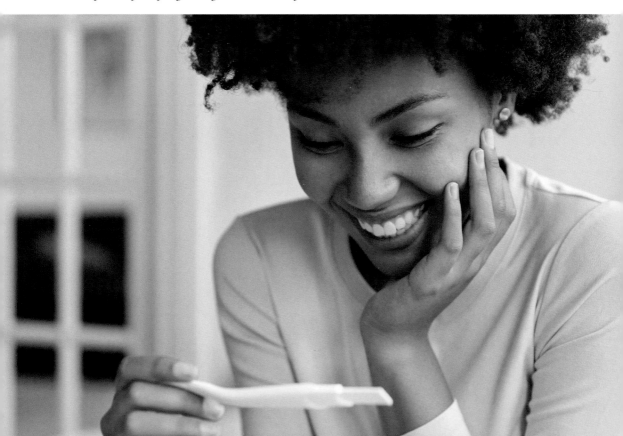

lower. The home pregnancy tests measure the level of a hormone, human chorionic gonadotropin (hCG), in your urine, and if the test shows positive it is unlikely to be wrong. It is possible to be pregnant and have a negative test result, but this generally happens if you have tested too early and you may need to repeat the test. There are also some types of medication that can affect the results, so read the leaflet in the box carefully if you are taking anything regularly.

One sign of early pregnancy most people know about is morning sickness, and it may be the first thing we expect to notice. In fact, morning sickness usually kicks in at around six weeks and although it is referred to as morning sickness, it can happen at any time during the day or night. Some women may feel nauseous rather than actually being sick. You may have a heightened sense of smell and some smells can become intolerable. Coffee, alcohol, nicotine and fried foods are often culprits. You may go off some foods too. Nausea and sickness can have a big impact on your daily life if you are badly affected. The other thing that is likely to make a difference to your life at this stage is tiredness and the idea of any kind of exercise routine in the early days of pregnancy may be unappealing, regardless of whether you are usually active.

It will take some time for your pregnancy to be visible to others. In the early days, your breasts may feel tender or swollen and the veins on the breasts may stand out more. Your nipples may be very sensitive or tingly and the skin around them may darken. You may need to pass urine more frequently and may be constipated. Some women have a strange taste in their mouth in early pregnancy which is sometimes described as being sour or metallic. You may notice an increase in vaginal discharge. The changing hormones of pregnancy can also lead to mood swings. While some women will experience lots of these early signs, others may not notice any significant changes at all. This is perfectly normal so there is no need to worry if you don't have the symptoms you were anticipating.

It can be frustrating if you want to keep fit to find your early pregnancy is dominated by feeling sick or exhausted. Don't forget that the sickness and tiredness will usually fade away by the end of the first three months, so you can afford to give yourself some leeway. It is a good idea to listen to your body rather than trying to push yourself to do too much, and gentle exercise such as walking can be a good way to keep active without over-exerting yourself. Many women find they have more energy as the pregnancy progresses.

MEDICAL CARE IN PREGNANCY

Once you know you are pregnant, you will need to make a medical appointment through your GP or local midwifery service so you can start the antenatal medical care you will receive throughout your pregnancy. You may have a first appointment where they will run through some basic information, followed by a more

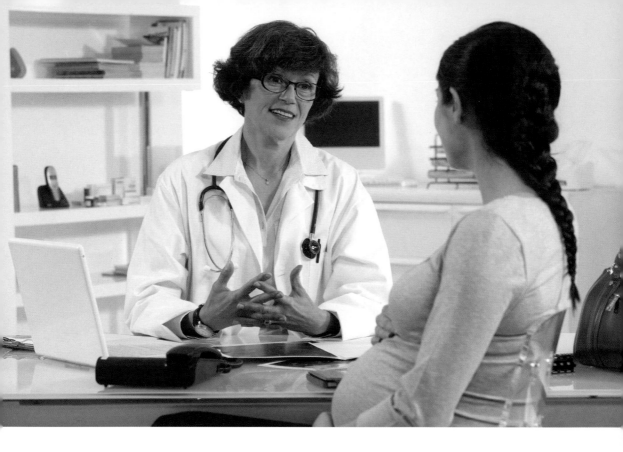

comprehensive appointment at around eight to twelve weeks. This appointment, sometimes known as a booking appointment, should cover key aspects of pregnancy including exercise, nutrition and diet and will explain the care you will receive and screening tests you will be offered. Your height, weight and blood pressure will be measured. You will probably have a urine test and a blood test to check your blood group. This test will also check for anaemia, which is common in pregnancy and is usually caused by a lack of iron. You may be asked about any previous pregnancies, miscarriages or terminations and about your family medical history. This appointment is also likely to include some discussion about your options for giving birth, breastfeeding and maternity benefits. It may seem premature to be considering these things so early in your pregnancy, but it is a good idea to have plenty of time to think about what is important to you.

Most antenatal appointments will be with a midwife. If there is any reason to assume the pregnancy may be more complex – for example, if you are expecting more than one baby or have an existing medical condition which may impact on your pregnancy – you may see a doctor. This would usually be an obstetrician who is a specialist in pregnancy and birth.

The number of antenatal appointments you have depends in part on whether there are any problems with the pregnancy; if all is going well you are likely to be seen less frequently. Generally there are fewer appointments in the first months, with more regular antenatal checks from twenty-four weeks of pregnancy. During these checks, your doctor or midwife will want to know about you and your baby. They may check your weight and ask for a urine sample which may be tested for infection, glucose (to check your blood sugar level for signs of diabetes) and protein (which can be a sign of a condition called pre-eclampsia later in pregnancy). They may also calculate your baby's growth by measuring the distance from the top of your womb to your pubic bone and listen to the baby's heartbeat.

Most women have at least two ultrasound scans during pregnancy: one between eight and fourteen weeks and the second at around eighteen to twenty weeks to check your baby's physical development. These are screening tests and look for conditions such as Down's Syndrome or physical abnormalities. You may also have blood tests as part of your screening and if there are concerns, further tests may be suggested. These tests, which are more invasive, look for genetic or chromosomal problems. You may be offered CVS (chorionic villus sampling) which is carried out between eleven and fourteen weeks and involves taking a sample of cells from the placenta, or amniocentesis, where a sample of the fluid surrounding the baby (amniotic fluid) is taken and analysed after the fifteenth week.

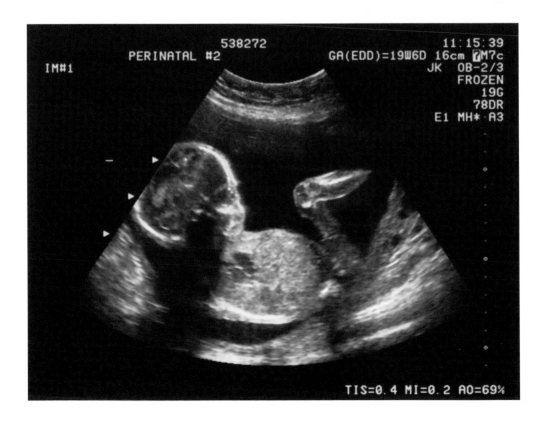

YOUR CHANGING BODY

Your body may not noticeably alter shape in the early days of pregnancy, although you are likely to be aware of changes, and the point at which your pregnancy starts to show to other people will be different for every pregnant woman. You will probably find that your breasts swell before you notice your tummy growing.

Inside your body, the fertilized egg or embryo implants itself into the lining of the womb. The cells of the embryo divide and multiply, and the outer cells link up to your blood supply while the inner cells begin to develop into the baby. The embryo has a small yolk sac in the early days which nourishes it but as it grows, a placenta is formed which is attached to the lining of the womb and joined to the baby by the umbilical cord. It filters oxygen and other nutrients from your blood supply for the baby. The inner cells form layers and these will become the different parts of your baby's body. Little buds appear where limbs will grow and gradually more of the organs will develop.

Usually by the end of the first three months, your tummy will be rounder and you will have started to be aware that you are losing your waist. Your clothes will feel tighter around the middle and you are likely to have gained some weight unless you have experienced severe morning sickness. It may take another month or so before you start to become obviously pregnant to other people.

By the start of the second trimester, the baby has grown to about the size of a peach and is starting to look more like a person. The bones grow harder and stronger and by the end of the fourth month your baby even has fingernails. By the final trimester,

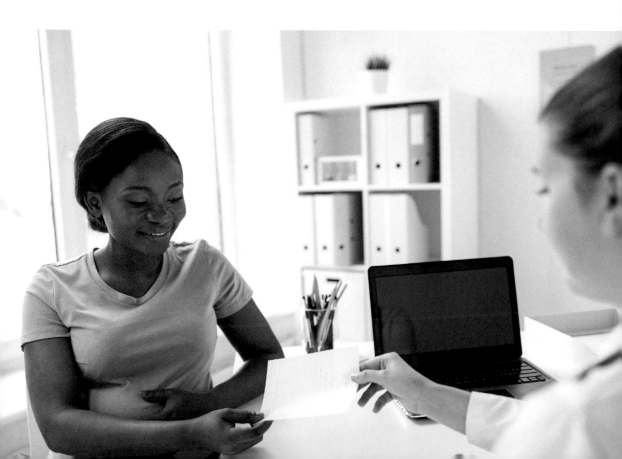

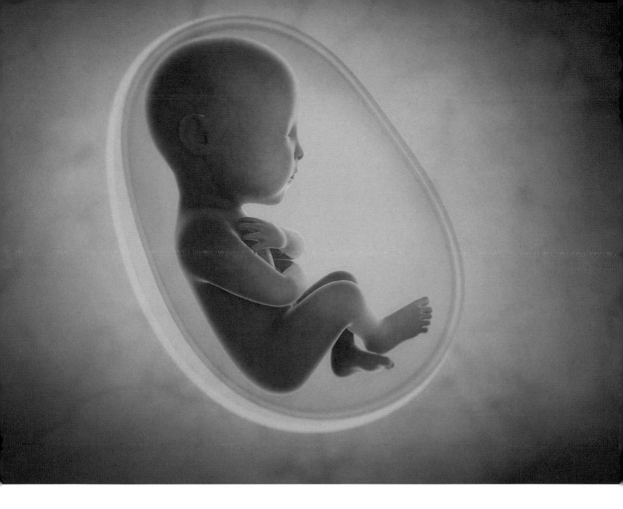

your baby is already quite well-developed and is starting to get ready for life outside the womb: the lungs prepare to breathe, eyelids open and fat builds up under the skin so the baby becomes plumper and rounder.

There are ligaments on each side of the womb which stretch, becoming longer and thicker as the baby grows. Usually your womb is about the size of a small pear, but at the end of the first three months it has grown to about the size of a grapefruit and by the time your baby is born it is the size of a watermelon, so these ligaments have a lot of stretching to do. Sometimes this can be uncomfortable and if you move suddenly or cough or sneeze, you may feel a sharp pain on one side. This is known as round ligament pain and is most likely to happen in the second trimester.

During pregnancy, your womb expands out and up, filling your abdomen. Women often worry whether they are growing at the right rate during pregnancy and you may not seem the same size or shape as someone else who is expecting a baby at the same time, but this is normal. Other people may have an opinion as to whether you are 'too small' or 'too large' for your dates, but it is best to discuss any concerns you may have about your size with your midwife or doctor rather than with well-meaning friends.

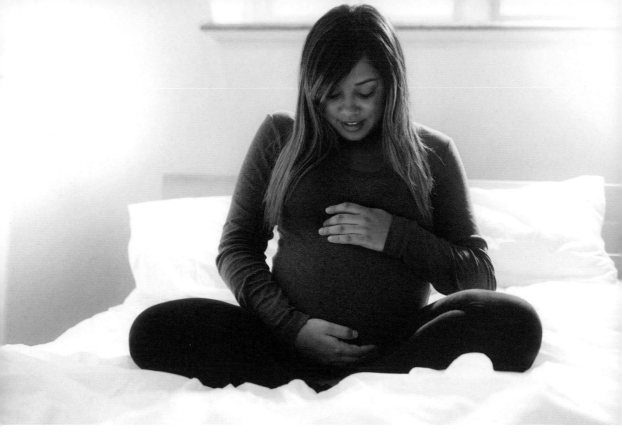

As your baby grows bigger and heavier towards the final few months of your pregnancy, your tummy keeps growing too and you are likely to experience more physical symptoms. Your increased weight, hormonal changes and the shift of gravity in your body as you expand outwards can make you feel really big and quite uncomfortable in the last few weeks. You will slow down too as it becomes more of an effort to be active.

HORMONAL CHANGES

In early pregnancy, the first change in hormones in your body is the production of human chorionic gonadotropin (hCG), which helps your body to prepare for a baby. Your levels of hCG start to go up early in pregnancy when the embryo implants into the lining of the womb and increase very quickly during the early weeks. This is the hormone that pregnancy tests check to see whether or not you are pregnant.

During your pregnancy, the levels of oestrogen and progesterone in your body will be higher than usual. Initially, you produce these hormones yourself but once pregnancy is established the placenta starts producing oestrogen and progesterone. You need lots of oestrogen and progesterone to help your body support the growing baby and to increase your blood supply.

You also have more of a hormone called relaxin in pregnancy, which relaxes your body ready for giving birth. It is responsible for softening the ligaments and muscles in your body. Some women feel a loosening of joints during pregnancy, and this can lead to aches and pains. You may find that your feet grow a little bigger and this is due to relaxin which loosens the ligaments in your feet. Coupled with your increased weight, this can cause the bones in your feet to spread.

Hormonal changes can affect your teeth too, which are at greater risk of plaque when you are pregnant. Inflammation may result from this and some women experience sore and bleeding gums when they are expecting.

Higher oestrogen levels and an increased blood flow to the vagina can lead to changes in vaginal discharge. You may notice more discharge in pregnancy and as long as it is similar to the discharge you would normally see during your cycle, there is usually no reason for concern. Talk to your midwife or doctor if you have any worries about discharge.

BREAST CHANGES

The first physical change that you may notice during pregnancy is a swelling of your breasts as they start to adapt for breastfeeding. Most women find they grow by one or two cup sizes during pregnancy, which may or may not be welcome. Your breasts may feel tender, and your nipples may stick out more and look darker. Towards the very end of pregnancy, your breasts may leak a little colostrum, a thin yellow liquid which is the first milk your baby drinks after birth.

CHANGES TO YOUR URINARY SYSTEM

Needing to pee more frequently is a common pregnancy complaint. This is partly because hormonal changes mean that blood flows more quickly through your kidneys, which makes them produce more urine. As your womb grows and puts pressure on the bladder and the pelvic floor, this can lead to stress incontinence and you may leak a little urine if you sneeze or cough.

CHANGES TO YOUR POSTURE

Your posture changes during pregnancy to allow you to carry so much additional weight in your abdomen. Backache is common as your centre of gravity changes as your womb grows.

CHANGES TO YOUR SKIN

Not everyone gets stretch marks during pregnancy, but the majority of women will. Stretch marks are indented streaks that appear on your skin as it stretches due to your increasing weight and changing shape. They are usually pink or red and are most often found on the legs, tummy and breasts.

You may also notice changes in the colour or pigmentation of your skin. Some women get darker patches of skin on their face and their nipples may also appear darker. Many women also get a dark line that runs down from the belly button to the pubic area. This is known as the *linea nigra* (Latin for 'black line') and it will usually fade away after the birth.

CHANGES TO YOUR DIGESTIVE SYSTEM

Constipation is very common during pregnancy as hormonal changes slow down the way your digestive system works. This can lead to another frequent complaint of pregnancy: piles or haemorrhoids. Piles are swollen veins that are found around the rectum or anus and they are caused by straining which puts pressure on the veins. They can be uncomfortable or even painful, but they usually go away naturally after you have given birth.

Hormone changes can also cause indigestion and as the size of your womb increases, it can push against your stomach and intestines and this can lead to heartburn and reflux.

Sickness and nausea are common signs of pregnancy and feeling sick is most common in the first three months of pregnancy. There is a condition called hyperemesis gravidarum which is a severe form of morning sickness in which you are unable to keep food down. Women who have hyperemesis can end up losing weight and becoming dehydrated, and may even need to spend time in hospital.

It is important to eat a healthy and balanced diet during pregnancy. Some pregnant women become anaemic which makes you very tired. This happens when the number of red blood cells that carry oxygen around your body is low. It is often caused by a lack of iron as the growing baby is using up some of your stores of iron. If you are anaemic you may be given a supplement as anaemia can lead to a higher risk of problems in pregnancy and after birth if it is not addressed.

CHANGES TO YOUR BREATHING

Your hormones can affect your respiratory system when you are pregnant, and women often say that they feel breathless. You need more oxygen for your baby and so you breathe more deeply, taking in more air. Later in pregnancy, your womb presses on your lungs and the muscle under them as your baby grows and this can affect your breathing too. If breathlessness becomes severe at any point, you should always seek urgent medical help.

GETTING READY FOR BIRTH

Towards the end of your pregnancy, your body starts to get ready for your baby to be born. Your baby's head may drop into the birth canal, but some women will go into labour without this ever happening. If your baby's head does drop, you may feel an increased pressure on your pelvis which can be very uncomfortable. It can also give you a tingling sensation, a bit like pins and needles, in the pelvic area from the pressure.

You may start to experience practice contractions. These are known as Braxton Hicks contractions after a doctor, John Braxton Hicks, who first noticed them in pregnant women in 1872. You may experience a brief tightening of your abdomen which may just last for a few seconds or can go on for a minute or two. These are not usually painful and you should talk to your midwife or doctor if you are having painful contractions.

You can read more about what happens when you give birth at the end of this book, but it is clear that the experience of pregnancy and birth can help us to appreciate quite how amazing the human body is. If you are fit and strong, this can help to make pregnancy and birth a smoother process, and looking after yourself will not only ensure that your baby has the best possible start in life, it will also help you to be in the best possible shape to care for your baby once he or she is born.

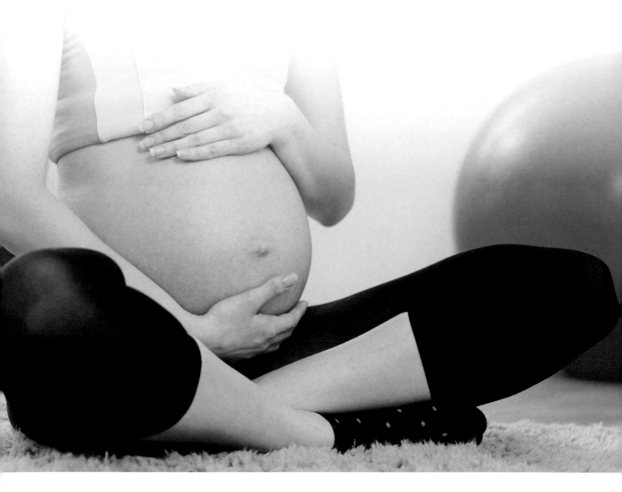

CHAPTER TWO

Nutrition for Pregnancy

Despite the large number of books, articles and websites devoted to the healthy pregnancy diet, there is really no great mystique to eating well in pregnancy. The guiding principles of a balanced diet that will help to keep you fit and well are pretty much the same for a pregnant woman as they are for anyone else, apart from certain foods you should avoid. Many women feel concerned about whether they should be eating more or less of certain foods, how much weight they should be gaining and what they should cut out. You may find that what you eat is to some degree governed by how you feel as nausea and sickness may limit your diet in the first few months and certain foods can become more or less attractive when you are pregnant.

During pregnancy, you have an opportunity to give your growing baby a good start through eating healthily. This does not have to be complicated, but is a matter of following the sort of diet we know we should be aiming for anyway. This means eating at least five portions of fruit and vegetables every day with the balance of starchy carbohydrates (such as rice, potatoes or pasta), dairy, protein and unsaturated fats (the sort found in olive oil or nuts and seeds). You should eat some protein every day

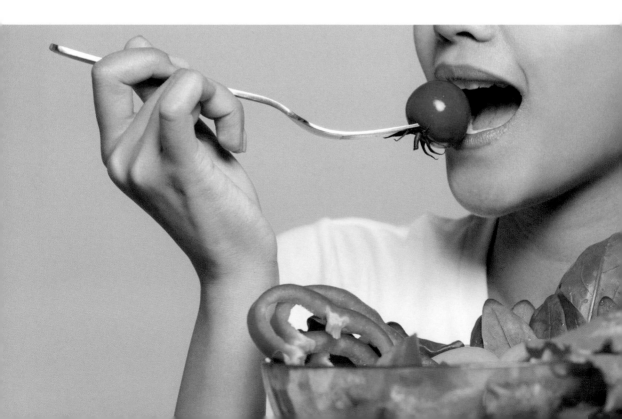

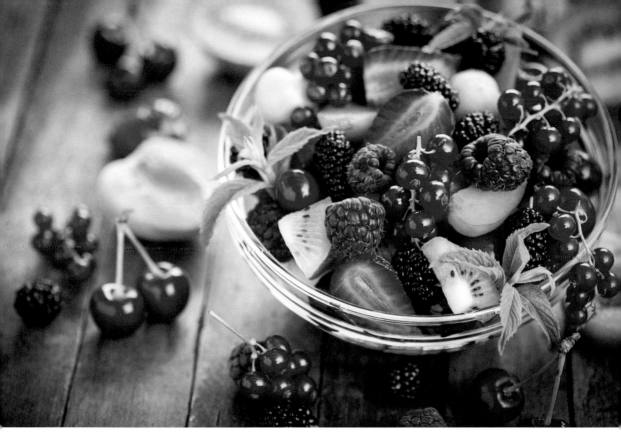

but that does not have to be meat; you can have fish, lentils, beans or tofu too. Try to choose wholegrain fibre-rich foods. This kind of balanced diet is more important than ever during pregnancy.

WHAT NOT TO EAT

There are some foods women are advised to avoid during pregnancy as these may have the potential to make you or your baby unwell. There are other foods you can eat in moderation but should avoid having in large quantities. Do bear in mind that most of this advice is precautionary, so it is focused on avoiding any potential risks for you and your baby. If you end up eating something you later realize you shouldn't have done or have eaten something on this list before you knew you were pregnant, there is no need to panic as it is likely that you will be absolutely fine. If you have any concerns or any symptoms you are worried about, discuss these with your midwife or doctor.

Cheese

Cheese is a source of calcium and vitamin B12. Both of these are important in pregnancy and most cheeses are fine to eat when you are expecting a baby. You can have any type of hard cheese, like parmesan or cheddar, even if they

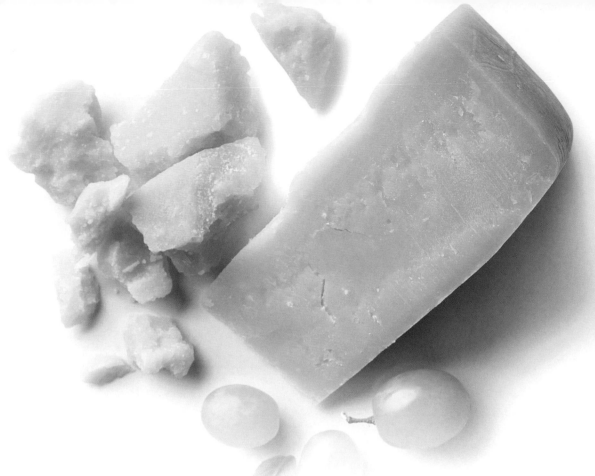

have been made with unpasteurized milk. You can also eat soft cheeses such as mozzarella, halloumi, feta, cottage cheese and cream cheese. What you should avoid in pregnancy are **mould-ripened soft cheeses with white rind**, for example brie, camembert or goat's cheese. The other cheeses to avoid are **soft blue cheeses** like gorgonzola or Danish blue. You can eat these soft cheeses if they have been cooked.

The reason for avoiding soft cheeses is that they can contain listeria bacteria which grow in moist conditions, and the infection you can get from this (listeriosis) is particularly risky in pregnancy as it could affect your unborn baby and could cause miscarriage or stillbirth. The symptoms of listeriosis are a bit like a mild type of flu and can include headaches, aches and pains, a high temperature, diarrhoea and feeling or being sick. If you think you could have listeriosis, your midwife or doctor may suggest a blood test to check.

Meat

You should not eat **raw or undercooked meat** when you are pregnant, so that means avoiding things like steak tartare and rare beef. Any meat should be cooked well, so it is no longer pink and there are no traces of blood. You should wash your hands after touching raw or uncooked meat, keep it separate from other foods in the fridge, and be careful to wash knives and chopping boards carefully too. This helps to guard against the risk of getting toxoplasmosis, which is caused by eating raw or undercooked meat that has been contaminated by a particular parasite. Although toxoplasmosis is very rare, it can sometimes damage an unborn baby during pregnancy and cause miscarriage or stillbirth which is why it is not worth taking any unnecessary risks. Toxoplasmosis does not always have symptoms, but people who have it may have a high temperature, aches, sore throat, nausea and swollen glands. If you have any concerns about toxoplasmosis, talk to your doctor or midwife.

Cold cured meats such as salami or Parma ham may also carry a risk of toxoplasmosis. These may have been smoked, dried or salted rather than cooked. If you cook these kinds of meats or freeze them for at least four days before eating this will prevent any risk, but you may wish to cut them out altogether. It is safe to eat ham or cooked meat that is pre-packaged.

One meat to avoid in pregnancy is **liver,** and that includes foods made with liver such as liver sausage or liver pâté. The reason for avoiding liver is that it is high in Vitamin A, and large doses of Vitamin A can be harmful to your baby. In fact, you should not eat any type of **pâté** when you are expecting as it can contain listeria, and that includes **vegetable pâté**.

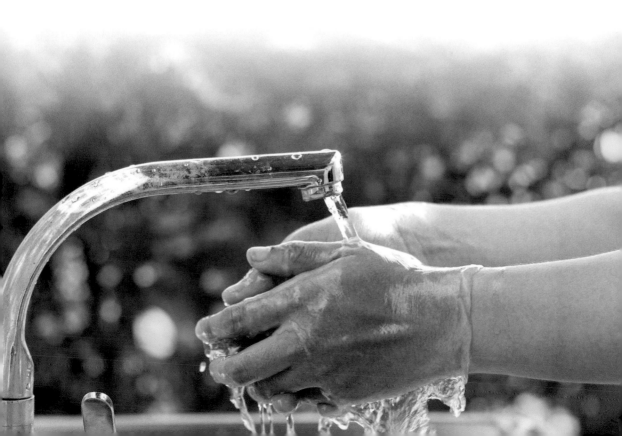

Eggs

For some years, the advice had been that pregnant women should avoid eating raw or partially-cooked eggs as there was concern that they could contain salmonella which can lead to food poisoning. The Food Standards Agency has now updated this advice to say that raw or lightly-cooked hen's eggs are fine if they are produced under the British Lion Code of Practice. This is a scheme that was developed to prevent salmonella, and the Code of Practice gives a set of standards which egg producers have to follow if they want their eggs to qualify. The majority of eggs that we eat in the UK are produced under this scheme, and you can check easily as all Lion Code eggs have a red lion printed on their shells. This means that things like mayonnaise and soft-boiled eggs are fine if they are made using Lion Code eggs. If you are eating out and you are not sure which eggs have been used, it is best to continue to avoid anything containing raw or partially-cooked eggs. Ice cream is usually fine but if it is home-made, make sure the eggs are Lion Code. Other types of egg should still be cooked thoroughly.

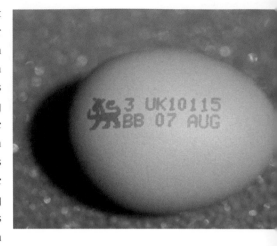

Unpasteurized Milk

The milk you find in supermarkets is pasteurized, but you may occasionally come across what is known as raw or unpasteurized milk for sale direct from milk producers or at a farmers' market. You are advised to avoid this in pregnancy. It will be labelled to say that it is unpasteurized so you are unlikely to consume it by mistake. You should also avoid unpasteurized goat's and sheep's milk too, and other products such as yoghurt that is made with unpasteurized milk.

Fish

Fish is a good source of protein and is a healthy food to eat in pregnancy, but there are restrictions on some types of fish. Oily fish, such as salmon or mackerel, is generally very good for you but can contain high levels of mercury so limiting your oily fish to two servings of fish a week is suggested as too much mercury could be risky for your baby. You should not eat more than two fresh tuna steaks weekly either, but if you are eating tinned fish you can have up to four medium-sized cans of tuna a week. Swordfish, shark and marlin contain more mercury than the other types of oily fish, so it is not advisable to eat them at all when you are pregnant. Eating raw shellfish, such as oysters, is not advisable because of the risk of food poisoning.

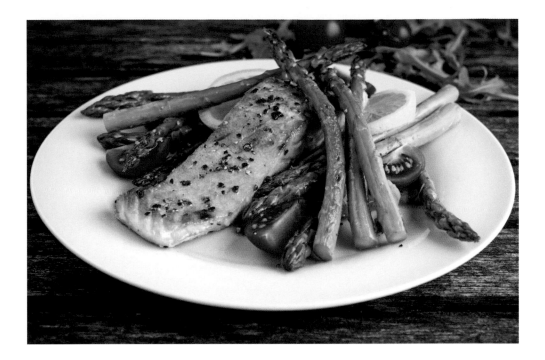

You can eat shellfish that has been cooked thoroughly, but some women find it easier to avoid shellfish altogether.

You should also be careful with **sushi** which is safe as long as the fish has been frozen for at least four days before being used (which is often the case with the type of pre-packaged sushi you may find for sale in shops). Sushi made with fish that has been smoked or pickled is all right too, but you should not eat sushi made with raw shellfish.

Caffeine

You can continue to enjoy a cup of coffee when you are pregnant, but if you are someone who usually fuels their day with espressos, you will want to keep an eye on how much caffeine you consume. Pregnant women are advised to keep to 200mg of caffeine a day but the amount of caffeine in your cup of tea or coffee can vary considerably depending on what you use to make it and how strong it is. The NHS advises that there is about 75mg in a cup of tea, 100mg in a cup of instant coffee and 140mg in a mug of filter coffee. There may be more variation than this as researchers from Glasgow University looked at the levels of caffeine in espressos from different coffee shops and found huge differences in a single shot from as little as 51mg of caffeine to as much as 322mg. There is also caffeine in cola (about 40mg per can) and energy drinks (80mg per can), and in chocolate (a 50g bar of dark chocolate is usually less than 25mg and the same amount of milk chocolate would usually be less than 10mg).

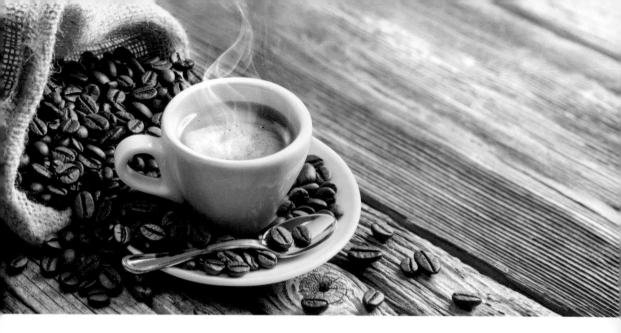

Occasionally going over the 200mg limit in a day is unlikely to be an issue, but very high levels of caffeine consumption have been linked to low birth-weight babies and miscarriage. If you enjoy tea and coffee, you may want to swap to decaffeinated and cut out energy drinks and cola altogether.

Women often swap to **herbal or green tea** during pregnancy, but the Food Standards Agency recommends no more than four cups of herbal tea a day when you are expecting as it says that there is no scientific evidence about the safety of these teas in pregnancy.

Alcohol

The most recent advice from the National Institute for Health and Care Excellence (NICE) is that women should avoid alcohol entirely in the first three months of pregnancy, and should drink no more than two units of alcohol once or twice a week for the rest of the pregnancy. Many of us are not entirely clear what a unit of alcohol is, and it may come as a surprise to learn that a large glass of wine in a pub or restaurant can contain three and a half units of alcohol and even a small pub glass of wine is usually more than a unit. The number of units in a drink depends on the strength of the alcohol as well as the quantity, so a pint of beer is often said to be two units but may be three if you are drinking a stronger brew. When it comes to spirits, a single pub measure tends to be no more than one unit.

You may find that you don't feel like alcohol when you are pregnant anyway, but when you do drink, your baby drinks too as alcohol passes through your blood to the baby's placenta. When women drink to excess in pregnancy, this can lead to miscarriage and premature birth. Sometimes the baby can develop fetal alcohol syndrome, a serious condition that causes learning and behaviour problems, poor

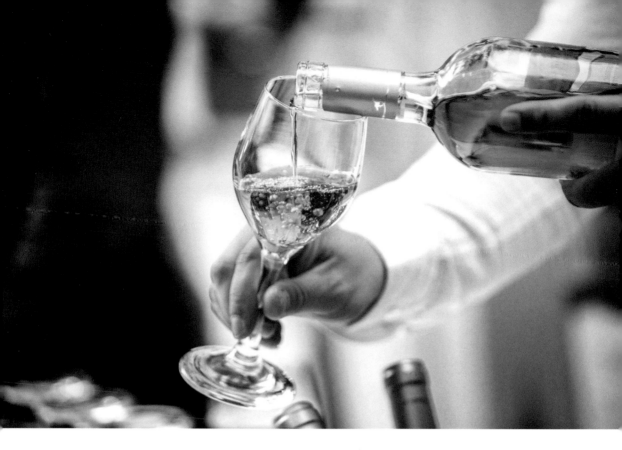

growth and can affect the way a baby looks, causing facial abnormalities. Having an occasional glass of wine when you are pregnant is clearly not going to lead to this kind of problem, but being mindful about your alcohol consumption is wise.

Sometimes women are very worried about the alcohol they drank in early pregnancy before they realized they were pregnant, but the reality is that most women don't know they are pregnant from the moment they conceive. Unless you were drinking very heavily and regularly, this is unlikely to have harmed your baby. Your midwife or doctor will be able to advise if you are concerned, but it is more important to focus on ensuring you don't drink more than is advisable for the rest of your pregnancy. If you are having difficulty stopping drinking and think you may have a problem with this, seek advice as soon as you can as medical professionals can help to ensure you get some support.

HOW MUCH WEIGHT SHOULD YOU GAIN DURING PREGNANCY?

Women are often uncertain how much weight they will gain during pregnancy and whether they will be able to lose it afterwards. It's important to be clear that there is no absolute 'right' amount of weight that a woman should gain in pregnancy and no formal evidence-based guidance on this in the UK. Despite this, you will probably find various figures for what is thought to be an estimated average weight gain, but

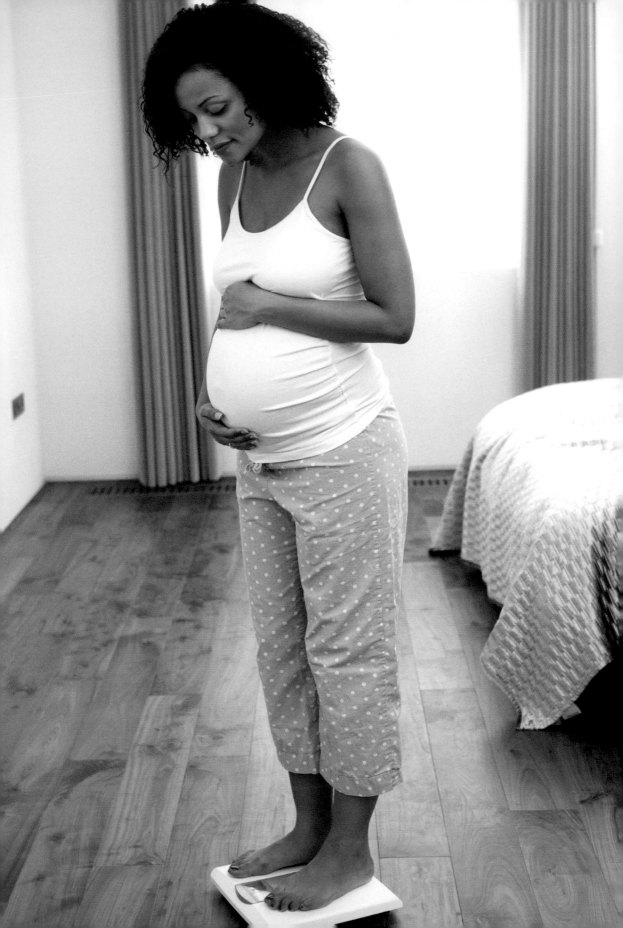

do remember that these figures are always averages. The amount of weight you gain is very much dependent on your height, pre-pregnancy weight and the size of your baby as well as on how much you eat and exercise during your pregnancy. You can be very healthy and gain more or less than average.

If keeping in shape has always been very important to you, the idea of watching yourself grow bigger in pregnancy may feel slightly alarming, but gaining weight is an inevitable part of pregnancy. You are carrying your growing baby as well as the baby's support system. The placenta that feeds the baby and the sac of amniotic fluid that surrounds the baby will add to your weight. Your womb itself is heavier as it becomes more muscly and you have more fluid and blood than usual in your body. Your breasts, which will have swollen, will also weigh more. Quite apart from this, you need to gain some extra fat which your body stores during pregnancy to help you to breastfeed your baby. This is not the time to go on some kind of weight-loss regime, but rather to eat healthily and sensibly to ensure that your baby gets all the nutrients he or she needs. There is an increased risk of prematurity and a low-weight baby if you don't gain sufficient weight in pregnancy.

You may have an idea that you will need to eat a lot more when you are expecting, but the old adage about eating for two during pregnancy is far from true. The number of extra calories you need each day during pregnancy is surprisingly low: according to NICE, a pregnant woman does not need additional energy supplies until the last three months of pregnancy and even then you should only be consuming an extra 200 calories a day. If you find that you are ravenous during pregnancy this guidance may seem

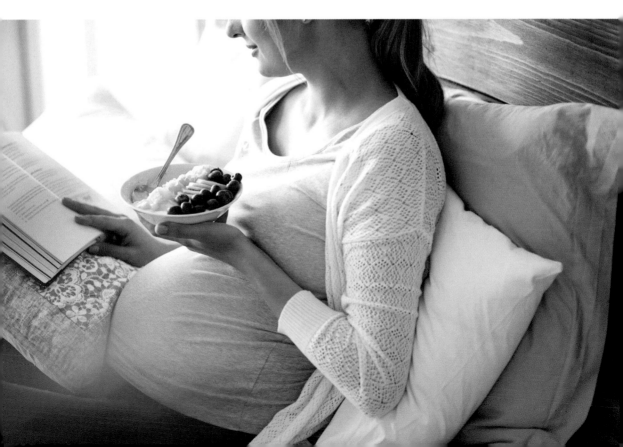

rather confusing, but cutting out unhealthy food and focusing on good nutrition will allow you to eat more without hugely increasing your calorie intake. Sometimes there can be a temptation to think that it is fine to have as many biscuits or cakes as you like because you are pregnant and although there is no harm in eating these things from time to time, your baby needs healthy food rather than empty calories. One study found that a third of pregnant women said that they experienced a loss of control over eating during pregnancy and these women tended to gain more weight and were more likely to have children who went on to become overweight. If you do put on an excessive amount of extra weight when you are pregnant, it's not just a concern because you may find it harder to lose it afterwards but also because it can affect you and your baby with a greater risk of high blood pressure, of pre-eclampsia and gestational diabetes.

You may be weighed when you have a check-up during your pregnancy and your weight gain will be monitored. Usually most of the increase in weight takes place during the second half of pregnancy but if your midwife or doctor has any concerns about your weight gain, they will discuss this with you. If eating is a problem during pregnancy, either because you are eating too much or finding it hard to eat enough, talk to your doctor or midwife as they can then offer more tailored advice and support.

CRAVINGS IN PREGNANCY

You may have heard about women who develop strange cravings when they are pregnant and become obsessed with eating lumps of coal or other usually inedible substances such as chalk or burnt matches. This is known as *pica* and it is quite unusual but if you find yourself with an urge to eat things that are not edible, don't hesitate to talk to your midwife or doctor about it as it is clearly not a good idea to be eating coal or chalk.

What is more common is to find that your tastes change, so foods or drinks that you usually enjoy become less appealing and you develop cravings for something you have not been particularly bothered about in the past. We are often told that we should listen to our bodies when it comes to food cravings in pregnancy, but if you find you have an overwhelming desire for daily doughnuts, this is probably not one to follow. If, on the other hand, you suddenly crave carrot juice or spinach, there is no reason not to have more of them. As long as your cravings are not desperately unhealthy, listen to what your body is telling you.

VEGETARIAN AND VEGAN PREGNANCY

If you are a vegetarian or vegan, you are likely to be told at some point during your pregnancy that you need to eat meat or fish or dairy produce to have a healthy baby. The truth is that many vegetarians and vegans have perfectly healthy pregnancies,

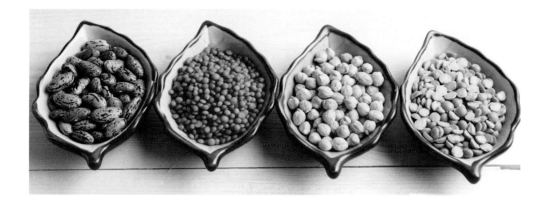

although they aren't eating meat, fish or dairy. Being a pregnant vegan or vegetarian does mean that you may need to think a bit more carefully about your diet during this time. The key things you need to ensure you are getting enough of are iron, vitamin B12, vitamin D and calcium, as well as plenty of protein.

You can get iron from dried fruit, pulses, wholemeal bread, leafy green vegetables and fortified cereals. If you are a vegetarian, eggs are also a source of iron. Vitamin B12 can be found in fortified cereals, fortified soya drinks and in yeast extract (Marmite). Vegetarians can also get vitamin B12 from cheese, milk and eggs. Calcium is easy for vegetarians who can eat dairy foods. For vegans, calcium can be found in leafy green vegetables, pulses, bread, dried fruit, tofu, sesame seeds and tahini, along with the fortified soya, rice and oat drinks that you may use to replace milk.

If you are a vegan or vegetarian, you also need to ensure that you get enough protein when you are pregnant. For vegans that means things like tofu, pulses like beans or lentils and nuts and seeds, and for vegetarians that can include eggs and dairy foods too. If you are a vegetarian or vegan and want to discuss your diet in pregnancy, your doctor or midwife will be able to help you decide whether you should consider taking any supplements.

SICKNESS IN PREGNANCY

It is all very well to know about nutrition and what you should and should not be eating during pregnancy, but with 80 per cent of women experiencing some level of nausea and sickness in early pregnancy, your diet may be limited more by what you can face than by what you know you ought to be eating. It is most common in the first trimester of pregnancy, and morning sickness is not in fact limited to mornings but can strike at any time of day.

Feelings of nausea can be brought on by your sense of smell which often becomes more acute during pregnancy. Certain smells may make you feel sick, whether that's frying onions or someone wearing strong aftershave on the train to work. About half of pregnant women are actually sick, but many others experience nausea. Although it usually eases off as the pregnancy progresses, it can continue and some women develop hyperemesis gravidarum, a severe form of sickness which may require hospital treatment.

If you are experiencing morning sickness, there are some tips that may help to relieve symptoms. Eating regular small meals every two or three hours rather than three large meals a day is often recommended, and bland carbohydrates like crackers, oatcakes, bread, baked potatoes, rice and pasta are usually easier to tolerate than anything sweet, spicy or greasy. If you feel sick when you wake up in the morning, allow yourself plenty of time to get up and if you can bear to try something bland like an oatcake right away, this may help to relieve the nausea. Once you know which smells are particular triggers, you can try to avoid them. Eating cold food can help as you don't have the accompanying cooking smells. Make sure you drink plenty of water to prevent dehydration. Tiredness and stress can exacerbate the symptoms of pregnancy sickness, so get as much sleep as you can. Ginger is often recommended for women who are experiencing nausea, and you may want to try ginger biscuits or ginger tea to see whether that helps. Women sometimes worry that their baby will not be getting the nutrients it needs if they keep being sick, but babies are surprisingly good at taking what they need first.

If bland foods, regular eating and lots of sleep are not leading to any improvements and you are still having real problems keeping anything down, you should see your GP and midwife, particularly if you notice your urine is dark or you barely need to pee during the day. For women who are diagnosed with hyperemesis gravidarum, this can lead to dehydration, weight loss and low blood pressure. You may be given some form of medication to try to help with the sickness, but if you are still being very sick you may need to be admitted to hospital to be given intravenous fluids. Although this is a horrible condition to live with in pregnancy, it is unlikely to harm your baby.

SUPPLEMENTS

If you go into any health food shop, you will find rows and rows of different vitamins and supplements aimed at improving a whole range of health problems and at preventing others. For pregnant women, there is clear guidance about some supplements you should take and about others that are not suitable in pregnancy. You should not need dozens of different supplements, but there are some that are specifically recommended for pregnant women.

Folic Acid

All pregnant women should take a daily folic acid supplement during the first twelve weeks of pregnancy. It helps reduce the risk of what are known as neural tube defects, such as spina bifida, which can happen when the baby is developing. It may also help to reduce the chance of your baby having heart or limb problems and some brain tumours that can happen in childhood.

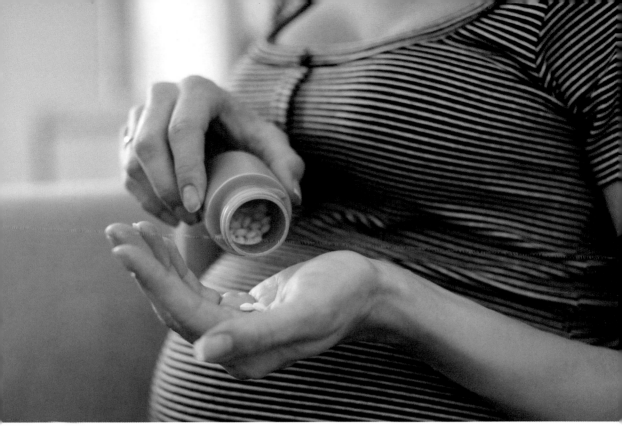

Folic acid is a B vitamin found in things like leafy vegetables and wholegrain cereals, but just eating more of these won't guarantee that you have the levels you need when you are pregnant, so you should take 400 micrograms of folic acid as a supplement each day. Women are advised to start folic acid supplements as soon as they decide they want to try to get pregnant, but if you have not done this it is fine to start taking folic acid as soon as you know you are expecting.

Women who have certain medical conditions that could increase their chances of having a baby with spina bifida are advised to take a higher dose of folic acid. Your doctor would tell you if you needed an increased dose and this may happen if you are taking some epilepsy medication, if you have coeliac disease, diabetes, sickle cell anaemia or thalassaemia, if you are very overweight, if you or your partner have spina bifida, if you have a family history of spina bifida or if you have had a previous pregnancy in which the baby was affected by spina bifida.

Vitamin D

Women who are expecting are now advised to take a daily supplement of 10mg of vitamin D during pregnancy and when they are breastfeeding. Our bodies make vitamin D when bare skin is exposed to direct sunlight when we are outside in the summer, but in the UK many of us have low levels of vitamin D, especially during the winter. If you spend a lot of time indoors, always cover your skin when you go outside and use sun cream, if you are overweight or if you have dark skin (for example, if your family is of South Asian, African, Caribbean or Middle Eastern origin), you are more likely to have low levels of vitamin D. This also applies if you have a diet which is low in the foods such as eggs, red meat, oily fish, cereals that contain vitamin D and margarines which are fortified with vitamin D. Sometimes if you are in one of these categories it may be suggested that you should take a higher than average dose of vitamin D, but your doctor will tell you if you need to do this. Taking a vitamin D supplement may also improve your baby's growth after birth and make it less likely that they will get rickets, a condition that affects the way bones develop, making them soft and weak.

Multivitamins

Some women choose to take a multivitamin, one pill or capsule that contains a range of different vitamins, when they are pregnant. You can get pregnancy multivitamins that have all the vitamins you need and are safe in pregnancy. They usually have some vitamin C to help the absorption of iron, and may have the folic acid and vitamin D that you need as well as a selection of other vitamins. If you are going to take a multivitamin, make sure you don't take a standard one containing vitamin A as this can be risky for your baby. You are also advised not to take high-dose multivitamins.

Pregnancy multivitamins can be pricey and the only elements of them you need when you are expecting are the folic acid and vitamin D, so don't feel you have to take the multivitamins just because they are specifically marketed towards pregnant women.

Iron

Iron supplements can irritate your stomach and lead to constipation or diarrhoea, so only take them if your doctor or midwife has prescribed them. They may be suggested if your iron levels are low and you are suffering from anaemia which can make you feel very tired. You can always try to get more iron from your diet; lean meat, dried fruit, leafy green vegetables and nuts are all high in iron. Some breakfast cereals have added iron too.

SUPPLEMENTS THAT ARE NOT RECOMMENDED

Vitamin A

Women who are pregnant should not take vitamin A supplements. High levels of vitamin A can affect the way your baby's nervous system develops. This is why you are told to avoid liver and liver products like pâté when you are pregnant as they are rich in vitamin A.

Fish Liver Oil Supplements

It is fine to take supplements made from the body of the fish (omega-3 supplements) when you are pregnant but you should not take supplements made from fish liver oil (such as cod liver oil). Again, this is down to the fact that fish liver oil supplements may contain high levels of vitamin A.

CHAPTER THREE

A Safe Pregnancy

When you are pregnant, you will want to avoid any unnecessary risks but you may find you are faced with conflicting evidence about what is and what is not safe for pregnant women, particularly if you start trawling the internet. Although online information can be very helpful, there is also quite a lot of misinformation and inaccurate advice. Unless you know it is from a reliable source, it is always best to take advice from your midwife or doctor if you have any uncertainties about whether you ought to be doing something or not.

OVER-THE-COUNTER MEDICINES

We are used to buying medicines from a local pharmacy or chemist to deal with day-to-day health issues such as headaches or sore throats, and we often take over-the-counter remedies without really thinking about what they contain. Some of these are fine to take when you are pregnant, but others are not and it is always advisable to check. Your pharmacist, midwife or doctor will be able to give you advice on which over-the-counter medicines are suitable to take in pregnancy.

If you are experiencing any discomfort that you would usually medicate, such as a mild headache, stop and think whether you really need a painkiller or other medicine.

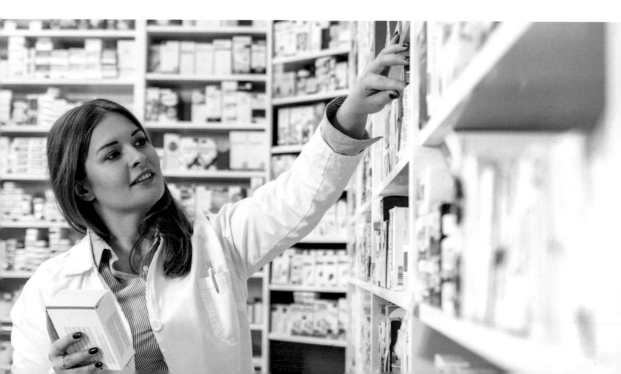

Of course, this does not mean you should spend the day with a blinding headache just because you are pregnant, but equally you don't want to take any medicines on a regular basis during pregnancy without some discussion with a healthcare professional.

PAINKILLERS

Most of us resort to taking some kind of painkiller now and again if we are experiencing mild to moderate pain. Check with a pharmacist, your midwife or doctor that what you are planning to take is safe in pregnancy as some types of painkillers carry more possible risks for pregnant women and their babies than others.

Paracetamol

This is often seen as the safe painkiller to use in pregnancy, but there have been recent concerns about whether taking paracetamol when you are pregnant might have some impact on your child in the future. The advice from the NHS is that paracetamol is usually safe to take in pregnancy but, as with any medicine in pregnancy, you should take the lowest dose that is effective for the shortest time. There are some paracetamol pills that may be labelled as 'extra' or 'plus' which contain caffeine and they are not recommended as you should be limiting your caffeine intake while you are pregnant.

Ibuprofen

If you want to take a painkiller in pregnancy, paracetamol is usually advised rather than ibuprofen. Ibuprofen has been linked to an increase in risks during pregnancy, including miscarriage, so it is generally advised that you should avoid it when you are expecting. If you have taken ibuprofen before realizing you were pregnant or in the earlier stages of pregnancy, it is unlikely to have had an impact on the baby but if you have taken it after thirty weeks of pregnancy, talk to your midwife or doctor.

Aspirin

Some women are prescribed low-dose aspirin during pregnancy, for example those who are assessed as being at high risk of pre-eclampsia or women who have a condition that increases their chances of getting blood clots during pregnancy. If you have been prescribed aspirin during pregnancy, this is because it has the potential to make a difference for you. If you have no medical reason to take it, it is best to avoid aspirin while you are pregnant.

HAY FEVER REMEDIES

If you suffer from hay fever, you know how unpleasant the sneezing, snuffling and itchy eyes and nose can be. Some over-the-counter hay fever remedies are all right to use in pregnancy and others are not, so check whether the type of treatment you prefer is OK to take when you are expecting. Pregnant women are sometimes recommended nasal sprays as a first hay fever treatment. Some types of antihistamine tablet are safer than others during pregnancy so it is a good idea to make an appointment to see your doctor if you feel you need antihistamines as they will be able to offer advice on this.

PRESCRIPTION DRUGS

If you take any regular medication, check with your doctor to find out whether there are any issues with it during pregnancy. If you are still at the stage of planning a pregnancy and you take regular medication, it is a good idea to get advice before you become pregnant. If you are already pregnant and you are on medication, the general advice is that you should not suddenly stop taking anything you have been prescribed, but should instead see your doctor about it as soon as you possibly can.

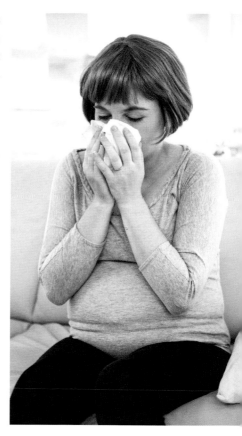

If you see a healthcare professional during your pregnancy about anything other than your pregnancy, make sure they know that you are pregnant before they prescribe anything for you. This will help them to work out how best to treat you and may alter what they choose to prescribe.

RECREATIONAL DRUGS

It will not come as a surprise to learn that you should not be taking any recreational drugs during pregnancy. Illegal drug use is widespread, and figures released in 2017 showed that around one in twelve adults had taken drugs in the last year. Using drugs in pregnancy carries additional risks for your baby as whatever you take may pass through the placenta. If you have been using any recreational drugs on a regular basis and worry you may struggle to stop, see your doctor or midwife as soon as you can. Don't feel embarrassed about this as being honest is far better for you and your baby. If those caring for you are aware of any possible issues, they can help you to get the right sort of support.

'Drugs can damage your baby and have the potential to cause a range of developmental problems and abnormalities. Smoking cannabis is often seen as so everyday that people imagine it does little harm, yet it is associated with lower birth-weight babies and may also affect your baby's brain development which can lead to long-term difficulties. Cocaine can cause abruption in which the placenta separates from the womb too early, which can lead to heavy bleeding and stillbirth. It may also affect the baby's brain and may lead to issues with learning and behaviour. Heroin may slow down your baby's growth and lead to premature birth. Babies who are exposed to heroin, cocaine and benzodiazepines in the womb can become addicted to them and when they are born they may have severe withdrawal symptoms.

SMOKING

It will really make a difference to your baby if you smoke while you are pregnant. When a woman who is expecting inhales the smoke from a cigarette, it contains thousands of chemicals that go straight into her lungs. Many of these chemicals can get into the woman's bloodstream and through the placenta to the baby. Cigarettes contain carbon monoxide and smoking reduces the baby's oxygen supply which can then increase their heart rate.

Smoking during pregnancy also brings an increased risk of miscarriage, low birth weight and premature birth. If you give up smoking, you reduce the risk of problems in pregnancy and birth, of stillbirth and of cot death. Your baby is also less likely to be born with certain birth defects. Even giving up smoking when you are already pregnant can make a real difference as most of these additional risks will be avoided if you stop in the first fifteen weeks.

It is not just your own smoking that affects your baby. If your partner or anyone else who lives with you is a smoker, this can also lead to lower birth weight and cot death, and can increase the chances of your baby getting bronchitis and pneumonia when they are born.

People who give up smoking cigarettes often turn to e-cigarettes, but it is not yet clear what impact the vapour from these can have on you and your baby during pregnancy. Although they don't contain as many chemicals as normal cigarettes, there may still be some toxins in the vapour you inhale from an e-cigarette. There should be support to quit smoking when you are pregnant through your local NHS Stop Smoking Service and you can find out more about the help you may be able to access from your doctor or midwife. Some people use nicotine replacements such as nicotine gum, patches or lozenges when they want to give up but this is not usually advisable if you are pregnant unless you have tried and not managed to give up without this kind of help. Talk to your doctor or midwife before using any kind of nicotine replacement.

ENVIRONMENTAL HAZARDS

Whether it's fragments of plastic in the fish we eat, toxic particles in the air we breathe or hormones in drinking water, there is growing interest in the role the chemicals we come across in our everyday lives may play in our health and this is likely to be of particular interest during the nine months of pregnancy. Concerns have been raised about a whole array of different products from household cleaners to pesticides, toiletries and food packaging. Most will have passed safety regulations and the impact of any one single product is likely to be small, but it is the build-up of the wide range of different things we come into contact with every day that some believe may be an issue. It would be impossible to lead a normal life avoiding every product that may carry an environmental question mark and there are many things you can't change, but if you are concerned about this you may want to consider taking some steps to reduce your overall exposure to toxins.

One of the key areas people often focus on when they think about environmental hazards is the residue from pesticides that may be found on fruit and vegetables, so pregnant women are advised to wash them before eating and to consider opting for organic. There are actually quite strict regulations about pesticide residues in non-organic foods, so it would always be better to carry on eating non-organic fresh fruit and vegetables in pregnancy rather than reducing your intake in an attempt to cut your exposure to any residues.

What we tend not to think about is the packaging our food comes in, but cans and other containers may contain chemicals that could potentially leach out into our food. Some food packaging can contain the chemical bisphenol A (BPA), and tiny amounts of this could be transferred from the container to the food. This sounds very alarming, but expert advice from the Food Standards Agency concludes that the levels of the chemical in cans and tins are not thought to be harmful and that humans quickly detoxify it and get rid of it from their bodies anyway. If you would rather avoid it, using fresh foods where you can is one way of reducing your exposure, and some women may choose to cut back their consumption of foods that are cooked in plastic containers.

Many everyday household products from oven cleaners to insect sprays carry warnings for their safe use and when you are pregnant you should make sure to read the advice on the labels and follow it. If you can, avoid using pesticides or fungicides (things like weedkillers or flea sprays) altogether. Women are sometimes concerned about fumes from household paint too, and although the risks of harm may be low, if you are having a room decorated you should make sure it is well ventilated and you may want to consider using water-based paints rather than solvent-based ones. Avoid turpentine, paint strippers or products that contain polyurethane, such as floor varnishes. If your job involves regular contact with solvents or substances you feel may be toxic, discuss this with your midwife or doctor and with whoever is responsible for health and safety in your workplace.

Concerns have also been raised about personal care products such as cosmetics and toiletries. Using these products is so much a part of our daily life that when we moisturize our skin with pleasantly-scented creams or use shower gels or scents, we may not always think about what they are made of, or about the fact that what we put on our skin may be absorbed into it. Women sometimes turn to products that are labelled as 'natural' or 'green' during pregnancy, but that does not guarantee that they are free from any chemicals. There are no regulations about what a product has to contain or not contain to be labelled in this way, and sometimes they may have additional ingredients that are not listed on the label. It is important to stress that there is no evidence that any individual product carries a risk and you do not need to stop using cosmetics and toiletries because you are pregnant.

While you are pregnant it is advisable to avoid having X-rays. The place this is most likely to arise is if you are having a dental check-up, so make sure you tell your dentist you are expecting a baby.

TRAVEL

Having a holiday before your baby comes along is always a nice idea, but you may have some concerns about long journeys and about which countries are safe to visit. There is no reason not to travel when you are pregnant, but you do need to be more careful. Travel insurance is essential if you are travelling abroad and make sure your insurer knows you are expecting a baby. It is worth avoiding places where there is a high risk of malaria if you can, and pregnant women are also advised not to make any non-essential journeys to countries where there is a high or moderate risk of the Zika virus (a disease spread by mosquitos which can cause birth defects). Stick to bottled water if you have any concerns at all about the local tap water and be extra careful about what you eat to reduce the risk of getting traveller's stomach upset.

Travelling by Road or Rail
Generally there are not any additional risks from road or rail travel when you are pregnant other than potential discomfort. Travelling can be particularly tough if you

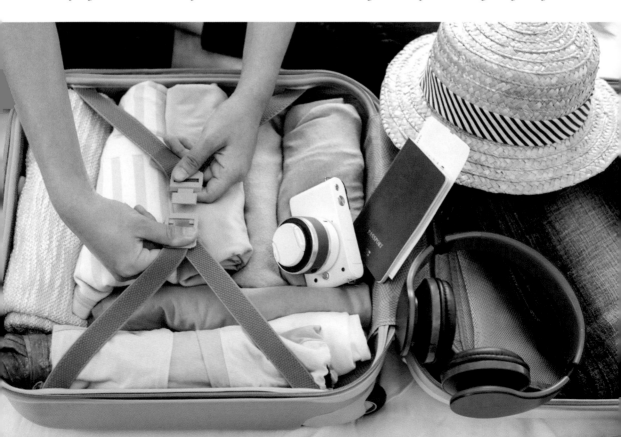

are feeling tired and sick in early pregnancy. In the later stages, sitting still for long periods can be uncomfortable and may make your feet swell and lead to leg cramps. Make things as easy for yourself as you can if you have to take long journeys in a car, coach or on a train. When travelling by rail or coach leave plenty of time to get to the station and for making any connections. Book advance train tickets with a seat wherever you can. Take water and some healthy snacks with you for the journey. If you are making a long journey by car, allow yourself plenty of stops along the way. There are no issues with driving when you are pregnant as long as this is not uncomfortable.

Travel by Air

As with road and rail travel, it is the discomfort of travelling by air which is the main issue with plane journeys for most of your pregnancy as long as there are no other problems. There are some medical circumstances in which flying when pregnant would not be advisable, for example if you have severe anaemia or a lung or heart condition, so it is always a good idea to discuss your travel plans with your doctor or midwife. In early pregnancy, flying can make sickness worse and your nose can get blocked and this may lead to problems with your ears. Check with your airline what their policies are before flying as once you get to twenty-eight weeks they may ask for a letter to confirm your due date and that you are safe to fly. Once you are in the final stages of pregnancy, at around thirty-seven weeks, most airlines will no longer want to carry you and this may kick in at thirty-two weeks if you are pregnant with twins, but different airlines have slightly different policies.

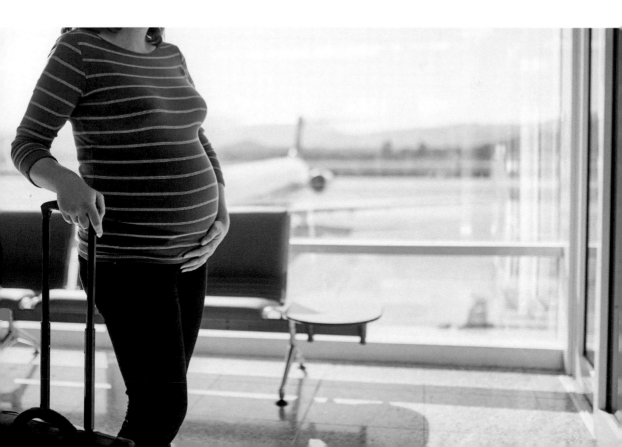

Blood clots are a potential problem for anyone on long-haul flights, but wearing compression stockings can reduce the risk. Make sure you get up and walk around a bit and there are also leg exercises you can do while sitting in your seat. Drink water during the flight rather than any caffeine or alcohol and wear loose, comfortable clothes.

VACCINATIONS

You may be concerned about having any vaccinations while you are pregnant, but there are some, such as the flu vaccine, that are fine during pregnancy. Women who are pregnant in the winter are recommended to have the flu vaccine as you are at higher risk of getting seriously ill from flu when you are expecting. You may also be recommended to have a whooping cough vaccination as getting vaccinated can help to protect your baby against the disease. It is fine to have a tetanus jab if you need one too.

The problem vaccines in pregnancy are those containing a live virus which you may need for travel to certain parts of the world. Vaccinations for yellow fever, oral typhoid and polio and the BCG vaccination for tuberculosis are not recommended in pregnancy, but if you cannot avoid travelling to an area where a particular disease is a risk, talk to your doctor about this. It is likely they will suggest having the vaccination anyway as this is usually much less of a risk than the disease itself. If you are travelling to an area where there is a malaria risk, discuss the type of protection you can take with your doctor as some are not suitable during pregnancy. There is a higher risk of getting malaria when you are pregnant because your immunity is lower. If possible, it is best to avoid travelling to places where you will need an array of vaccinations and protection against malaria when you are pregnant.

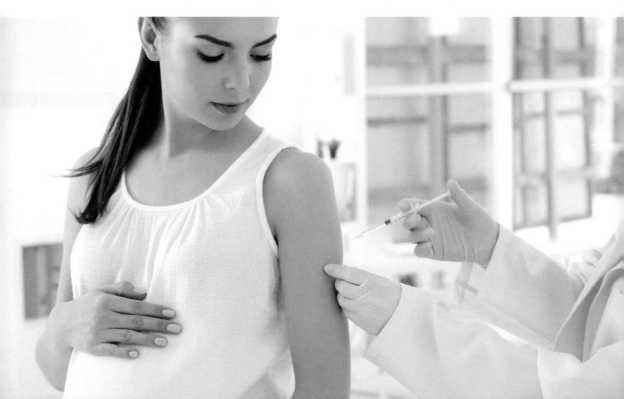

CHAPTER FOUR

An Introduction to Exercise in Pregnancy

We all know exercise is good for us and more and more women are reaping the benefits, whether that's from running, going to the gym, swimming, taking exercise classes or a wide variety of other activities. It is recognized that exercise can have a preventative role where our health is concerned, helping to protect us from disease and keep us fit and well. In the past, when there was the potential for so much more to go wrong in pregnancy, there was often a view that pregnancy was a delicate condition and being active might be risky. Although we know the evidence shows exercise is beneficial for the vast majority of pregnant women, there is still a lingering sense that keeping fit might be risky or even dangerous if you are expecting. What we don't always appreciate is that being active in pregnancy can have the same beneficial effect that it has at any other time of life and can help to prepare the body for the changes it will go through and for birth itself.

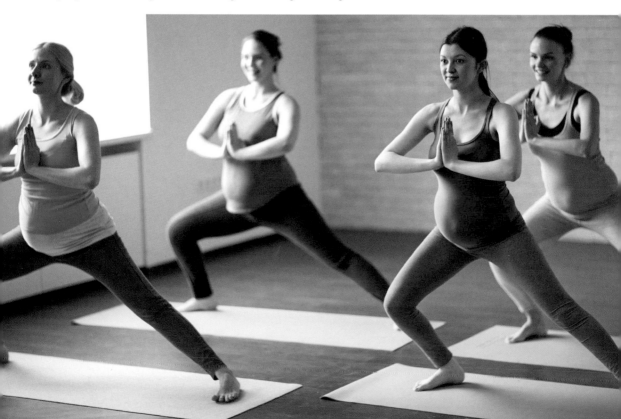

You are less likely to have back pain and muscle cramps, gestational diabetes and high blood pressure if you are fit, you will gain less weight and have better circulation. You may also have a lower risk of some common pregnancy problems such as constipation, leg cramps, varicose veins and bloating. Finally, you will be stronger and have more stamina and energy, better posture and balance and this can help you to be prepared for giving birth. A study from researchers at Madrid University found that taking regular exercise during pregnancy reduced the length of labour by some fifty minutes. You are also likely to recover more quickly after having your baby too, which helps to set you up for a more positive experience of early parenthood.

We often focus on these physical benefits, but the emotional benefits of keeping fit are just as important in terms of reducing stress or anxiety, increasing your energy levels and helping you to feel more positive, self-confident and happy. Exercise can help you to relax and to sleep better at night, which will have a positive impact on your overall sense of wellbeing.

If you have always exercised regularly, your interest may be in how best to continue this through the nine months of pregnancy. Keeping fit may have become part of your identity and you may be concerned about losing that if you can't do everything you have been used to doing. If the tiredness and exhaustion of early pregnancy means you feel less able to get to the gym, pool or track, this can make you feel physically and emotionally ill at ease. You may not be certain how much exercise you should take while you are pregnant and whether you will have to cut back.

If you haven't ever been into fitness, the idea of starting out when you've just found out you are pregnant may seem like very bad timing. This certainly isn't the moment to take up marathon training or body-building, but just being more active can be a positive thing for you and your baby. You don't need to have been a fitness fanatic in the past to reap the benefits and there are many gentle forms of exercise that will still be good for your body, boost your energy levels and help you to relax without making you feel uncomfortable or out of your depth.

Whatever your situation, exercise in pregnancy is all about what feels right for you. You do need to use some caution and you should never exercise if you are not feeling well or in very hot conditions. Also remember that you are not aiming to improve your speeds or achieve new personal bests but rather to keep active and healthy.

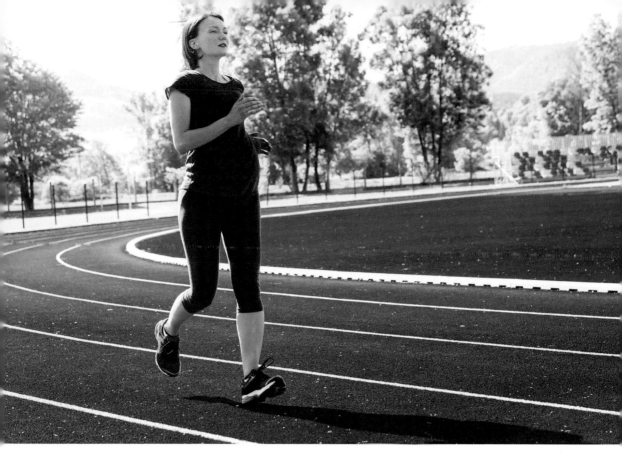

HOW MUCH EXERCISE SHOULD I BE DOING DURING PREGNANCY?

The only honest answer to questions about how much exercise you should do while you are pregnant is that there is no one response to this. The levels of exercise that are right for individual pregnant women are related to what you did before you found out you were expecting, to your fitness levels and your overall health. If you are a regular runner, someone is used to daily exercise classes or spending hours in the pool each week, what you can do while you are pregnant will clearly be very different to the levels of exercise advised for someone whose idea of keeping fit is walking to the bus stop.

There are a few key points about exercise in pregnancy that are relevant to everyone. The first is that it is always a good idea to discuss any exercise you are considering with your midwife or doctor when you are pregnant. They will know what is most suitable for you in relation to the levels of exercise you are used to and to your individual situation in pregnancy. It is also necessary to consider taking things a little more slowly and not to keep pushing yourself if you are starting to feel exhausted or uncomfortable. You should listen to your body. There are all kinds of different ways of keeping active and it is about finding what is right for you at any given point in your pregnancy as this will change over the nine-month period.

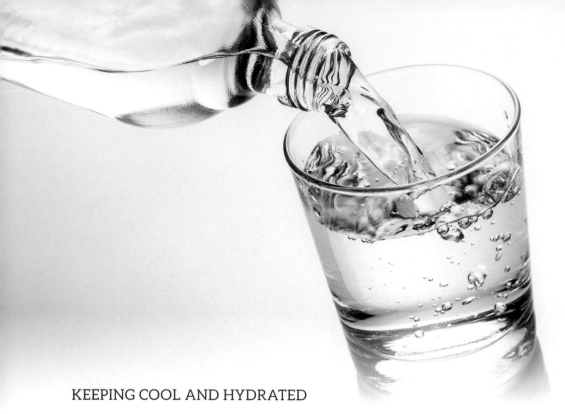

KEEPING COOL AND HYDRATED

If you are taking exercise while you are pregnant, you must make sure you are drinking enough fluids. Buy a water bottle and make sure you keep it filled up during the day as this will help you to avoid getting dehydrated. Always take water with you if you are out taking exercise. You should aim to drink at least eight glasses of water a day, but do this gradually spread out across the day.

You should also be careful not to get too hot when you exercise during pregnancy as your body temperature increases more than usual when you are pregnant. Don't push yourself too hard either, and be particularly cautious about taking anything other than gentle exercise in very hot or humid conditions.

PROTECT YOUR JOINTS

During pregnancy, your body becomes more flexible in preparation for giving birth and your joints become looser. This increases the risk of injury as the joints and ligaments are not as stable as usual. In order to ensure you exercise safely, it will help if you warm up first and cool down afterwards. Obviously if you are just going out for a walk there is no need to do a warm-up and cool down, but this does apply to any more intense exercise.

WHEN NOT TO EXERCISE

Although most pregnant women can exercise safely while they are expecting, you should always check your doctor or midwife is happy before starting any form of exercise. If you have what is labelled a high-risk pregnancy, perhaps because you are expecting more than one baby or because you have a pre-existing medical condition, you are likely to need to be more cautious about what kind of exercise you attempt and you may need to take it slowly and carefully.

There are some medical conditions that indicate you should not take up any kind of exercise until you have come up with a plan of what you can do with your doctor or midwife. These include the following:

- Anaemia
- Diabetes
- Epilepsy
- Heart disease
- High blood pressure
- Hyperthyroidism
- Lung disease
- Persistent bleeding
- Placenta previa
- Previous sports injuries
- Recurrent miscarriage
- Very low or high BMI

If you have any other medical condition and are uncertain about exercising in pregnancy, it is always advisable to err on the side of caution and discuss this with a medical professional. You should not be exercising once your waters have broken or if you have problems with your cervix opening early (cervical insufficiency).

IS THERE ANY EXERCISE I SHOULDN'T DO?

There are some forms of exercise that are not usually recommended in pregnancy. This tends to be when there is a higher than usual risk of falling over (such as downhill skiing) or exercises that could possibly involve your bump being hit (such as contact sports). Sometimes athletes who take part competitively in a particular sport continue when they are pregnant despite it not being recommended for most women, but these kinds of sports are usually best avoided for anyone else:

- Basketball
- Boxing
- Contact sports
- Diving
- Downhill skiing
- Gymnastics

- Hang-gliding
- Hockey
- Horse-riding
- Ice-skating
- Mountain-biking
- Rugby
- Surfing
- Volleyball
- Water-skiing

Caution is advised with other sports such as tennis and squash and after sixteen weeks you need to be careful about exercise that is carried out while lying on your back.

BEING OVERWEIGHT IN PREGNANCY

We know that being overweight is becoming more common and around a quarter of all women in England are classified as obese according to the Health Survey for England. This means that many of us are overweight when we get pregnant which can bring additional risks for both mother and baby. If you are overweight, you can make a difference to the progress of pregnancy, to the experience of birth and to recovery after having the baby by being more active in pregnancy.

If you know how much you weighed before you got pregnant, it may be helpful to work out your BMI (body mass index). You can find lots of online calculators to assess this for you and you just need to put in your height and weight. If your BMI is over 18.5 and under 25, your weight is healthy. If your BMI is over 25 but under 30, you are classified as overweight. If your BMI is 30 or more, this is classified as obese. It is important to do this with your pre-pregnancy weight as it may not be accurate if you have already started gaining weight in pregnancy.

If you have a BMI of 30 or more, you are at greater risk of getting diabetes in pregnancy and of pre-eclampsia, so those caring for you will be on the lookout for any complications. Pregnancy is not a time to go on a fad diet or follow a strict weight loss plan, but if you are overweight you should focus on eating healthily and taking exercise. If you haven't done any exercise before, don't worry as you don't need to start some kind of complex or gruelling exercise regime but just aiming to increase your activity levels in your day-to-day life will make a difference. Getting fitter will mean you are less likely to gain too much weight during pregnancy, which means you are also less likely to be left with a large weight gain after you have had your baby. Being more active will also increase your overall sense of wellbeing.

EXERCISE FOR THE INACTIVE

Some people find the whole idea of fitness very off-putting whatever their weight, and if the thought of going to a gym or wearing sports clothes fills you with horror, don't let that be an excuse to give up on being more active during pregnancy. You can get fitter without ever stepping inside a gym or a sportswear shop. There are lots of very simple ways to start to increase your exercise levels: use the stairs instead of getting in the lift, get off the bus a stop earlier and walk from there to your destination, go on foot to the shops instead of getting in the car, and if you have a very sedentary job where you are at a desk all day, make sure you get up every now and then and walk about for a few minutes.

If you don't see yourself as the exercising type and you are feeling exhausted in the early weeks of pregnancy, even this level of activity may seem too much. Once you are approaching the end of the first trimester, you are likely to find that you have more energy and being active may not be quite so uninviting. It is never too late to start, and exercising in pregnancy isn't about trying to turn yourself into some kind of super-fit athlete but rather about improving your overall health and wellbeing. Do have a chat with your doctor or midwife about exercise and what you would like to achieve.

If you haven't taken any exercise before or if you are overweight or obese, it is important not to suddenly start an extreme fitness regime but rather to gradually increase your levels of activity. You should initially start with no more than fifteen minutes of exercise three times a week if you have not taken regular exercise in the past and you can increase this slowly as it feels right for you. The aim is to reach half an hour of exercise four times a week, but anything you can reach working towards this goal is going to be beneficial.

Starting Out With Walking in Pregnancy

Walking is a great form of exercise to start with as you can go at your own pace, gradually building up to walking more briskly and a little further. You don't need any special equipment or clothing, just comfortable supportive shoes, and you can do it pretty much anywhere. Just being outside for some time each day will also help with your emotional wellbeing if you usually spend most of your day inside.

If you need some motivation for walking, you can always try to get friends or family to come along with you and go on a city walk or head out to the seaside or into the country. Don't forget to take water and a healthy snack with you if you are going on a longer walk as keeping hydrated is important. Unless you are a seasoned hill-walker, it is probably sensible to keep to relatively flat walks on level ground when you are pregnant; gentle hills are not a problem but you should still be able to hold a conversation when you are walking. A high-altitude scramble is not the sort

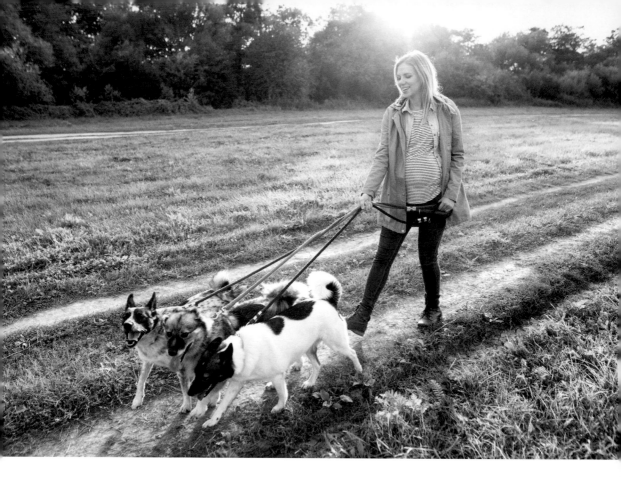

of thing you should be doing while you are pregnant unless you have experience of this kind of walking. During the summer always wear sunscreen, have some kind of hat or headscarf and avoid walking at the hottest time of day. You should also be careful about walking when it is icy outside in the winter when you are pregnant. You can walk right through your pregnancy but as you approach your due date, don't forget to take your mobile phone with you!

Starting Out With Swimming in Pregnancy

Swimming is another good form of exercise in pregnancy if you have not done regular exercise before or are overweight. It may be particularly beneficial in the last stages of pregnancy when other forms of exercise can become impractical as your weight is supported in the water. If you have a history of problems in pregnancy or medical conditions dating back before your pregnancy, you should talk to your midwife or doctor about exercise including swimming, but generally it is a safe form of low-impact aerobic exercise that tones your muscles and improves your cardiovascular (heart) health. You can do any stroke in early pregnancy but breast-stroke is often recommended as you get into the later stages, although it should be avoided if you have pelvic pain as breast-stroke legs may make this more uncomfortable. The one thing you should not be doing while pregnant is diving, particularly if your diving often ends up in a belly-flop!

Some local swimming pools run water aerobics or aqua fitness classes for pregnant women and these are great if you are not a particularly confident swimmer as most of the exercises are done in the shallow end of the pool. The exercises are designed for pregnancy and the classes also provide a good opportunity to meet other women who are expecting. You may find a variety of other water exercises on offer, such as Aqua Zumba which is dancing in water, and these are usually fine for pregnancy as long as you check with a medical professional and the instructor. A study from Brazil some years ago found that water aerobics classes were suitable for women with straightforward pregnancies even if they were not regular exercisers.

Some women are worried about the chlorine used to disinfect the water in public swimming pools and whether this can carry risks after a study reported that large amounts of a by-product of chlorine were risky for pregnant women and could increase the chance of their babies developing allergies later in life. The benefits of swimming in pregnancy are likely to outweigh any potential risk and the levels of chlorine in public pools are monitored. There would be a greater potential risk from swimming in pools without chlorine where there could be a danger of infection from contaminated water.

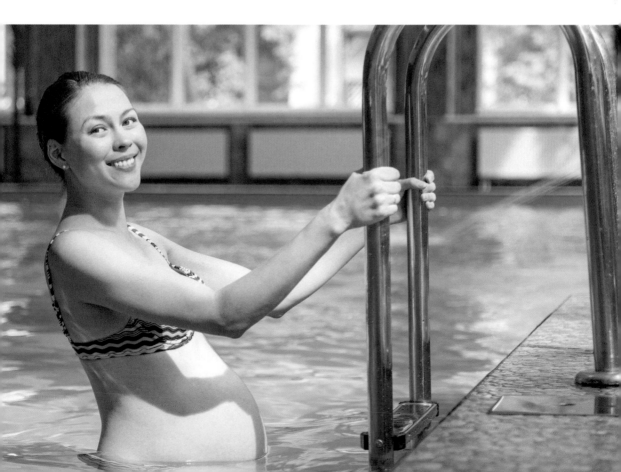

Starting Out at the Gym

If you haven't been to the gym before, you can start in pregnancy as long as you are careful. You must take advice about how to use the equipment properly and have an introductory session with a trainer who knows you are pregnant and who can discuss what is suitable for you to do. The treadmill, cross-trainer or stationary exercise bike may all be suitable when you are first starting out.

Starting Out With Exercise Classes

Not all classes at your local gym or fitness centre will be suitable for someone who has never done them before. Some, like spin classes which are high-intensity classes on an exercise bike, are really best for those who have pre-pregnancy experience. Others, such as aerobics or Zumba, may be possible if you take them at your own pace and talk to the instructor beforehand, making sure they know you are pregnant. If there are any fitness classes specifically aimed at pregnant women, these are often the best option for anyone considering joining a class for the first time when they are pregnant.

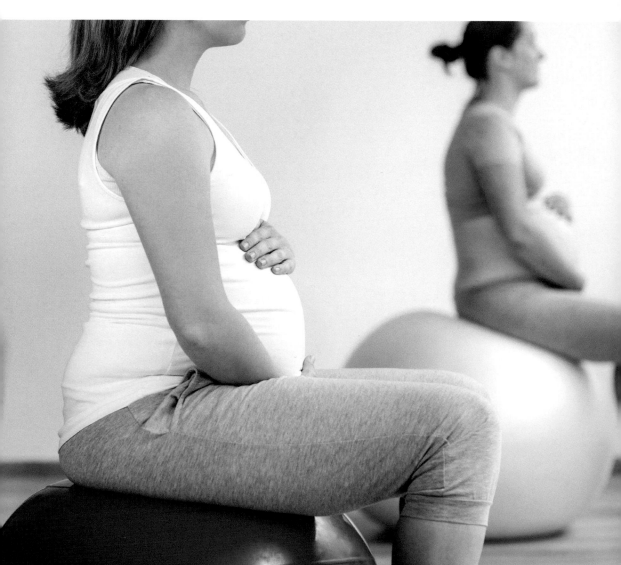

CHAPTER FIVE

Keeping Up Your Fitness in Pregnancy

Unless you are taking part in some kind of very high-intensity sport, there is no reason to completely give up on your fitness regime in pregnancy but many women find they don't feel up to what they are accustomed to during the first trimester of pregnancy. It can come as a shock to find yourself feeling debilitated if you are used to exercising regularly, but some of your usual energy will start to return once you are through the first stage of pregnancy.

Keeping active during pregnancy is good for you, but you need to be sensible and not over-exert yourself. You should listen to your body and adapt your expectations so you only do what you feel up to doing rather than pushing yourself in the way you might have done before you were pregnant. You can still feel challenged, but you don't want to carry on to the point of being unable to speak and dripping with sweat. You want to avoid getting overheated and keep yourself hydrated. You also want to be careful to protect your pelvic floor so if you are experiencing any continence problems in your pregnancy, talk to a medical professional or physiotherapist about the best exercise for you. While you are pregnant you may want to change the type of exercise you do, to cut back a bit and to always make sure you have a balance so that you are getting sufficient rest as well as taking exercise.

WALKING FOR FITNESS

Regular walkers may find they can carry on with quite long walks right up until they go into labour. This is fine as long as you take sensible precautions such as stopping to rest if you need to and taking lots of water and some healthy snacks as well as a mobile phone. Make sure you have the right shoes and clothing and avoid setting off on a long walk in the midday heat in the summer.

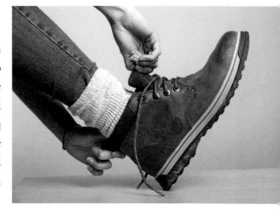

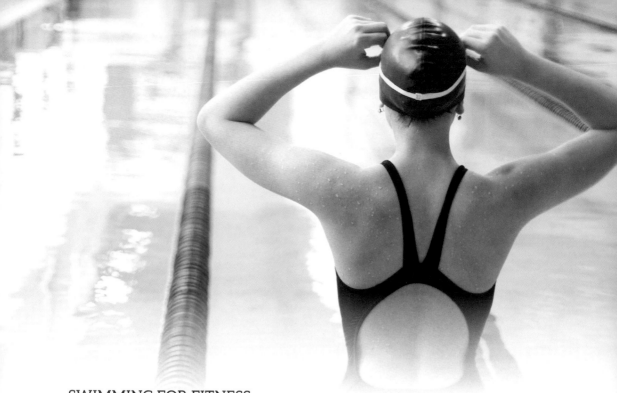

SWIMMING FOR FITNESS

This is often said to be the best form of exercise in pregnancy as the water helps to support your weight and you should be able to carry on as usual if you are a regular swimmer. You will probably find you start to swim more slowly and you will ease off a bit as you go through pregnancy. You may need to change strokes too, but unless there are any specific problems you should be able to carry on swimming throughout pregnancy. Tumble turns are usually all right at the start of pregnancy, but are likely to become uncomfortable as you get bigger and you will need to use the steps to get out of the pool too. Diving is not advisable during pregnancy, and you should also be careful about keeping hydrated and not getting too hot as you may not notice that you are overheating when you are swimming.

RUNNING FOR FITNESS

More than 2 million people in the UK are now reported to run on a regular basis, and although the advice in the past tended to be that running was not a suitable exercise during pregnancy, this is no longer the case. If you have a straightforward pregnancy without any problems and were fit and running regularly before you discovered you were pregnant, running is likely to be beneficial rather than potentially dangerous. A recent study concluded that babies born to regular runners who continued to run during their pregnancies were no more likely to have a low birth-weight or to be born prematurely. The important fact here, however, is that these women were used to running, which means they were more likely to be fitter and healthier than the

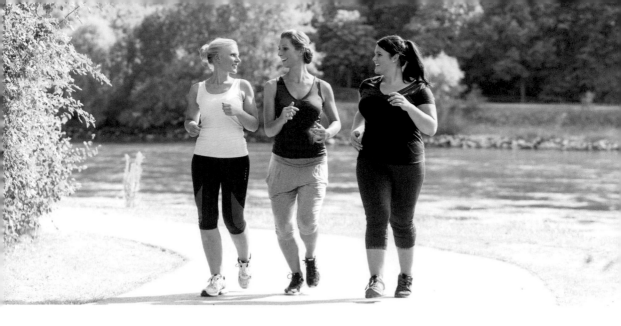

average woman. It is not the time to take up running if you've never done it before, and it is absolutely not the time to try to set a personal best or attempt a long run you haven't tried in the past.

For regular runners, the difficulty in pregnancy may be around accepting that over the next nine months you are likely to run more slowly and to run shorter distances. Talk to your midwife or doctor about your running – about what you are used to doing as part of your training and what you are planning to do during pregnancy – just to ensure that there are no concerns. If you are suffering from sickness and tiredness in the first trimester, you may not be up to running too much and you should always stop running right away if you start to feel dizzy or sick or have any other unusual symptoms. Sometimes this can mean that you get out of the habit, so you may need to start more gently than you would expect when you feel up to running again. Don't run when it is very hot outside, and make sure you take water with you as it is easy to become dehydrated. If you experience any problems relating to your pelvic floor, such as leaking or continence issues, you should always talk to your doctor, midwife or a physiotherapist about this rather than continuing to run as usual. One thing that is sometimes recommended in pregnancy is fartlek or interval training where you run faster- and slower-paced sections of a run, so you may do thirty seconds of running at pace followed by a minute of slow jogging. This can be a useful training option in pregnancy.

At some point running is likely to become uncomfortable and when that happens it is time to re-think and change your fitness regime. You may want to take up regular walking or swimming instead.

GYM FOR FITNESS

If you are a regular gym-user, carrying on with the treadmill, step machine, cross-trainer and exercise bike is fine in pregnancy. During the final stages of pregnancy you should take care if you are using a rowing machine, ski machine, climber or air walker. Having a chat with one of the instructors at the gym about which equipment is suitable for use in pregnancy will help you to work out a suitable routine.

WEIGHT-TRAINING FOR FITNESS

You need to approach this with some caution but you can do weight-training when you are expecting if you have done it before you were pregnant, have been instructed in how to use weights or any machinery properly in pregnancy and you make sure you are careful. Don't push yourself too hard and consider doing more repetitions with lighter weights rather than using weights you strain to lift. Lifting lying down and lifting weights over your head is not advisable as your pregnancy progresses. Talk to your instructor about modifying your weights regime during pregnancy.

BODY CONDITIONING FOR FITNESS

Some local gyms and fitness centres have body conditioning for pregnancy classes and these would be ideal. If you want to go to your normal class, tell the teacher you are pregnant and ask for guidance on which exercises to avoid. It is thought best to avoid exercises that involve lying on your back and don't do things on your tummy.

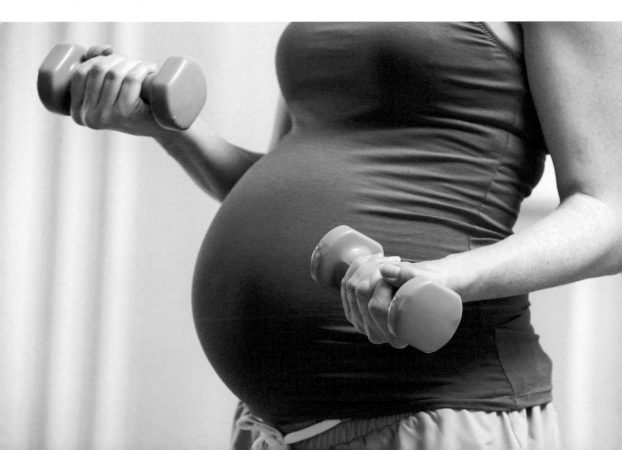

PILATES AND YOGA CLASSES

You will find more information about Pilates and yoga for pregnancy in the next chapter.

MARTIAL ARTS CLASSES FOR FITNESS

As with other classes, if you have done these before you were pregnant it is possible to carry on but you need to tell your instructor you are expecting. There will be some parts of the class you can't do and you should be cautious about physical contact.

STEP AND AEROBICS CLASSES FOR FITNESS

You can continue with step and aerobics classes if you have been doing them regularly in the past. Make sure the instructor knows you are pregnant as there are likely to be some parts of the class where they will give you an adapted exercise to try instead of what everyone else is doing.

SPIN CLASSES FOR FITNESS

These high-intensity cycling classes are not suitable unless you have done them before you became pregnant. If you have been spinning for some time, you can carry on but it is essential to make sure the instructor knows you are expecting. Do not expect to be able to go quite as fast, at the same level of resistance or for as long as you used to before you were pregnant.

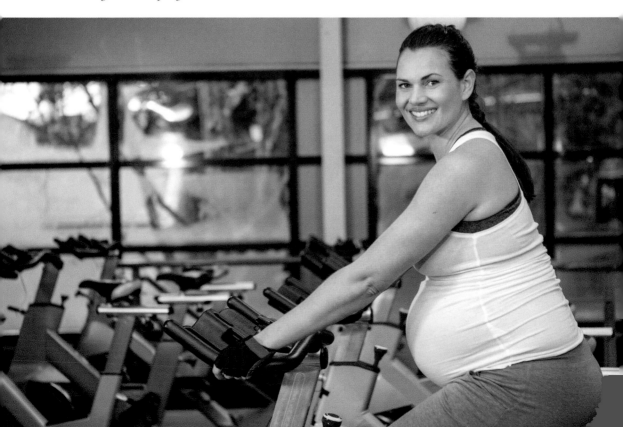

CYCLING FOR FITNESS

If you cycle regularly, you may find conflicting advice about whether this is safe during pregnancy with some experts warning against it because of the risk of falling while others maintain that it is safe. There is always a risk if you fall when you are pregnant, so you would need to take extra care but if you are keen to carry on cycling, you should discuss this with your midwife or doctor who will be able to assess your individual situation.

SIGNS TO STOP EXERCISING

There are some signs that show you should stop exercising:

- if you start to bleed
- if you start to leak amniotic fluid
- if you feel dizzy, faint or very breathless
- if you have a severe headache
- if your heartbeat is irregular or you have palpitations or pain in your chest
- if you feel contractions
- if you become suddenly exhausted
- if you have pain or swelling in your legs
- if you are experiencing shortness of breath
- if you have pain in the back, abdomen or pelvis.

If you experience any of these problems when you are exercising, you should stop right away.

CHAPTER SIX

Flexibility and Stretching in Pregnancy

Pregnancy fitness is not just about keeping active, but also about trying to keep flexible too. Regular stretching exercises can help with aches and pains in pregnancy and also keep your muscles toned. Your posture and balance are important too as your body adjusts to your growing baby and your centre of gravity changes.

If your growing bump is causing back pain, sciatica or pelvic pain, your midwife may recommend a pregnancy support band or maternity belt. These go under or around your bump and help to support your back. You are only meant to wear them for a few hours at a time rather than constantly, but they can be particularly helpful if you are out and about. Talk to your midwife about using a pregnancy support band or maternity belt as they may not be advisable if you have issues with your blood pressure or circulation.

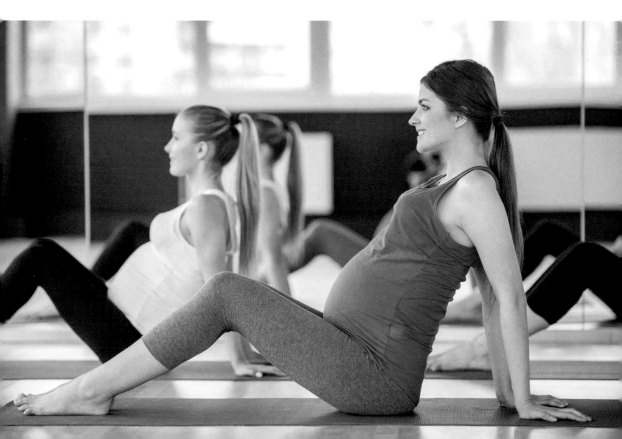

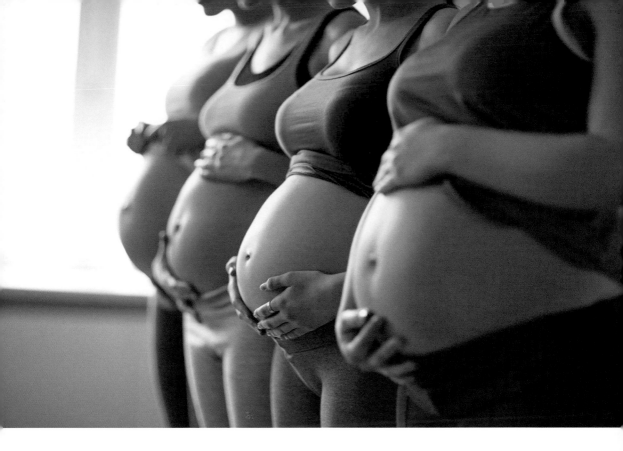

As your pregnancy progresses, sitting and standing properly with your back straight can help to prevent backache. You may need to use pillows to help with support when you are in bed as your bump grows, and sleeping on your side is best. Once you get to the third trimester, this is important as sleeping on your side reduces the risk of stillbirth. If you wake up on your back don't worry about this at all, but when you re-settle yourself back to sleep, do it on your side again. You can buy special pregnancy support pillows to help with your position when you go to sleep, or you can just put a normal pillow behind your back.

You should avoid heavy lifting and keep your back as straight as you can and bend your legs when you are picking anything up from the floor. If you are finding something too heavy, don't lift it but wait for someone else to help and when carrying shopping don't load it all on one side but instead balance it between two bags, one on either side. Wearing comfortable low-heeled and supportive shoes while pregnant will help too.

YOGA

Based on an ancient Indian philosophy, yoga is more than just physical exercise as it also uses breathing techniques and mindful relaxation. This can make it particularly beneficial in pregnancy as it is seen as a more gentle form of exercise focused on

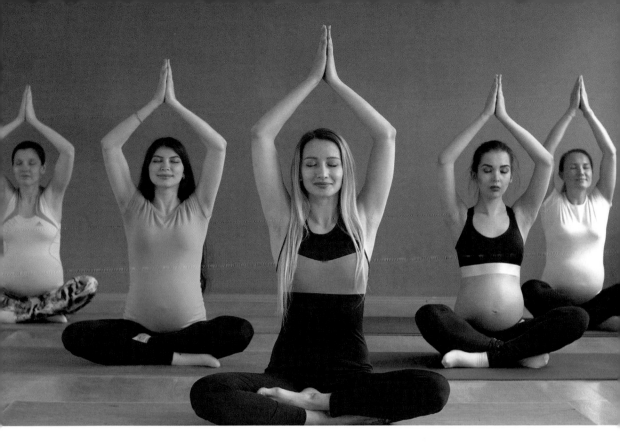

strength and flexibility. The breathing and relaxation techniques can reduce anxiety and may be really useful when you are in labour.

Antenatal yoga classes are very popular, and if you can find one near you this is a good way to start yoga if you have not done it before. The poses (known as asanas) in these classes are quite simple and the classes are put together specifically for pregnant women. You are generally advised not to do yoga in the first trimester if you have not done it before. Make sure your instructor is aware of any specific medical condition or pregnancy problems so you do not attempt anything that would not be right for you. If there isn't a pregnancy yoga class anywhere near you, you can join a general yoga class but there will be some asanas that are not suitable (such as certain twisting positions or inversions where you do shoulder-stands or headstands), so it is important to talk to the instructor about the fact that you are pregnant before you start.

Yoga is not an aerobic form of exercise but is focused on strengthening your muscles. You do not have to be fit or active to join a yoga class, but it can be surprisingly demanding. Yoga is never a competitive sport but should be about finding what works for you. There are many different types of yoga but the classes you should avoid when pregnant are Bikram or Hot Yoga which you practise in a hot, humid room as there are concerns about overheating and dehydration.

PILATES

Pilates is a system of exercise that aims to strengthen the body, making sure it is aligned properly. It helps with flexibility and improving your overall wellbeing and fitness. There is a focus on the core and Pilates is sometimes recommended for people who suffer with back pain. This means that it can be a good form of exercise during pregnancy when back problems are often an issue, and it can be helpful when your centre of gravity is changing as your body grows. Some Pilates exercises work on the pelvic floor and again this is great for pregnancy.

Pilates was originally invented by a German emigré, Joseph Pilates, who lived in England around the time of the First World War and later moved to the United States. He had a number of ailments as a child and was not terribly strong so he spent a lot of time trying to improve his physical strength. He researched different exercise regimes and eventually developed his own technique which he hoped would allow people to realize their full physical potential as he believed many were not as fit as they should be because of their lifestyles, poor posture and breathing techniques.

Most Pilates classes are done on a mat like a yoga mat, but sometimes you will find classes done on a Reformer, a frame with a platform on it attached by springs offering different levels of resistance. If you are experienced at Reformer Pilates you can continue with this in pregnancy, but as you progress through pregnancy you will need to change the way you use it so you don't lie on your back.

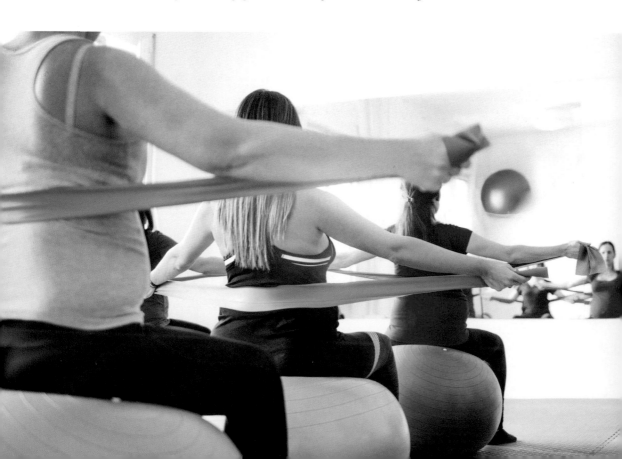

The best way to experience Pilates when you are pregnant is to join an antenatal Pilates class as there will be some exercises in a normal class that are not suitable during pregnancy. If there are no antenatal Pilates classes in your area and you have never done Pilates before, it is best to attend a class for beginners and make sure that the instructor knows you are pregnant.

THE MOST IMPORTANT EXERCISE OF ALL

Whatever else you do or don't do during pregnancy, there is one type of exercise every pregnant woman should continue on a regular basis and that is pelvic floor exercises. Your pelvic floor muscles hold your womb, bladder and bowels in place, help you to control your bladder and bowels and support the weight of your baby as it grows.

These exercises are important when you are pregnant because your pelvic floor is put under a lot of strain carrying your baby and during birth, and it will not be as strong afterwards. Pelvic floor exercises can help strengthen the muscles and reduce the risk of letting out urine involuntarily when you sneeze or cough (stress incontinence) which can happen when the pelvic floor muscles are weak. Having strong pelvic floor muscles will also help you to push your baby out when you are in labour and could shorten the second stage.

Women who have given birth vaginally are at greater risk of having a prolapse, in which the pelvic organs (bladder, bowel or womb) drop downwards into the vagina. This doesn't necessarily happen straight after you've had your baby, but may occur much later in life, often around the time of the menopause. Pelvic floor exercises can help to prevent this occurring.

Pelvic floor exercises are very simple to do: you just need to imagine that you are having a pee and need to stop suddenly. The muscles you can feel tightening are your pelvic floor muscles and you should be able to feel a sensation of pulling upwards and inwards. You should pull up slowly and hold the muscles tight and then release them; do ten or fifteen quick ones and then some slow ones where you hold the muscles tight and count slowly to ten before letting go. If you aren't sure you are doing your pelvic floor exercises correctly, talk to your midwife or doctor who will be able to give you more advice.

Sometimes women assume these exercises are only important just after they have given birth, but in fact they are best started in pregnancy and you should aim to continue them for the rest of your life as this will help to prevent problems of incontinence or prolapse that can happen during the menopause.

CHAPTER SEVEN

Your Emotional Health

Your emotional health may not be the first thing that springs to mind when you are thinking about having a healthy pregnancy, but it is just as important to your overall wellbeing as your physical health. During pregnancy your emotions can fluctuate as your hormone levels change and you may have unexpected worries, fears and anxieties. Pregnancy is a time of great change in every aspect of your life and it is inevitable that this will have some impact on your emotional wellbeing.

We expect pregnancy to be a time of great joy and happiness, but many women experience uncertainties and anxieties along the way, particularly with a first pregnancy, and this is perfectly normal. You may not be entirely certain that you really want a baby, you may not feel ready for motherhood and may be anxious about what lies ahead, you may worry about physical symptoms or whether your baby is growing as they should be, you may be concerned about what you should and shouldn't be doing when you are expecting. You may feel frightened about the prospect of giving birth or worried about being a good parent, and you can end up simply worrying about worrying.

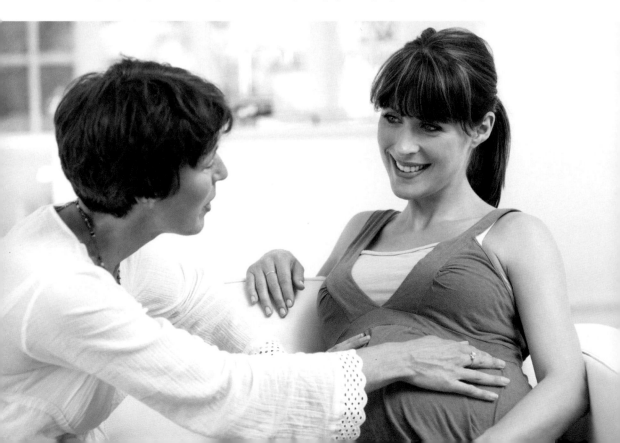

EMOTIONS IN EARLY PREGNANCY

In early pregnancy, it is very common to focus on pregnancy symptoms; whether that's symptoms you have that you aren't sure are normal, or symptoms you think you ought to have that you aren't having. One of the problems with so much information online is that everyone experiences pregnancy differently. We don't all have every symptom but it can be worrying if you start comparing your experience with that of other women. If you have concerns, it is always far better to raise them with your midwife or doctor, no matter how silly they may seem. Worrying about the baby and whether he or she is all right is a very normal part of being pregnant.

Being pregnant is life-changing and even if you were initially filled with delight or your positive pregnancy test, you may find that you have concerns about whether you are really ready for this and whether it is the right time to have a child. If you didn't intend to get pregnant, these uncertainties can be even stronger and it may take a while to adjust to the situation. Sometimes women worry that having conflicting feelings about their pregnancy is a sign something is wrong, but in reality thinking through these concerns can be integral to coming to terms with being pregnant and learning to embrace the changes that lie ahead.

YOUR CHANGING BODY

Many women have quite complicated relationships with their bodies when it comes to shape and size, and the idea of your body rapidly growing larger can be challenging. Although some women embrace the prospect of a pregnant belly, for others the thought of not being able to see their feet may be more troubling. Most of us have a mental image of what shape we should be and gaining weight does not always feel comfortable, especially if your body image has been very important to you. Perhaps the most difficult phase of weight gain during pregnancy is in the earlier stages when your thickened waist and swollen breasts may make you feel overweight rather than pregnant. As your pregnancy progresses, your shape gradually alters to accommodate your growing baby and you will be continually adjusting to this. Once you can feel your baby moving, it may be easier to start

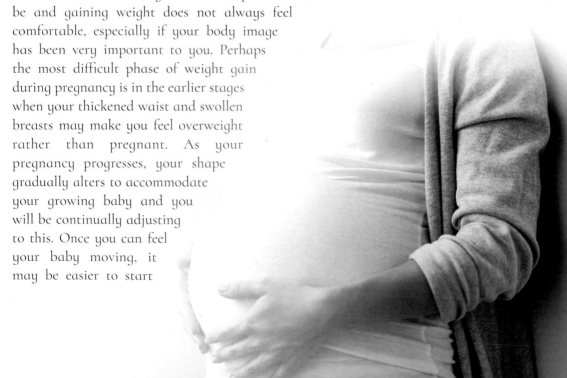

to focus your attention on their needs and to see your changing body as an integral part of a healthy pregnancy.

If you have had issues with your weight in the past or have suffered with an eating disorder such as anorexia or bulimia, you may worry about the impact of weight gain on your self-esteem. Some women find that being pregnant helps them to get over issues around food and weight, but this is certainly not the case for everyone. Don't feel embarrassed about telling your doctor or midwife if you have or have had an eating disorder. If gaining weight and being weighed regularly may be difficult for you it is important to make sure you have the right support.

RELATIONSHIPS

Being pregnant often puts a strain on relationships. This can be down to feeling tired or anxious, or it may be a sense that you are both dealing with pregnancy differently if it feels as if your life is already changing and your partner's isn't, or if your partner is not as focused on the pregnancy as you are. Your sex drive may change during your pregnancy too; some women find sex more enjoyable when they are pregnant but others find their libido decreases. This can have an impact on your relationship with your partner and talking about how you feel is important.

Sometimes there may be domestic issues that can affect your relationship with your partner during pregnancy; whether these are financial concerns about how you will manage for money once your baby arrives or perhaps practical problems around accommodation or employment. These can add to the burden of anxiety

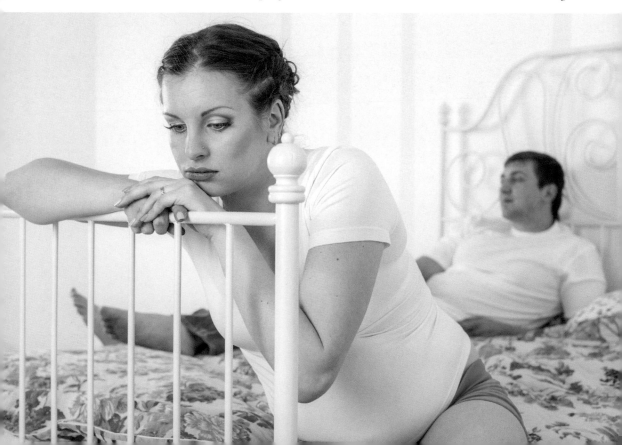

in pregnancy and can lead to disagreements or arguments. Conflicts can feel worse because you think you ought to be blissfully happy and contented if you have decided to have a family together. Understanding that this is can be a challenging time for any relationship as you both come to terms with what lies ahead may help to give some context to the situation.

DEALING WITH OTHER PEOPLE

One of the things you may start to notice when you are pregnant is that other people not only have views about pregnancy and birth, but may also be very keen to offer you their advice. Whether you have decided you'd like an epidural for pain relief in labour or you want a home birth with a birthing pool, if you are planning to go back to work soon after having your baby or want to give up work for a while to be a stay-at-home mother, there is likely to be someone who would like to tell you why you might want to think again.

Of course, this can be welcome if you are given practical tips for pregnancy and parenting, but what can be more difficult is advice that feels critical. Pregnancy can make you feel more vulnerable and you may question yourself if you are surrounded by people who seem to need to offer their views on what they think you ought to be doing differently. Women can start to doubt themselves and to feel overwhelmed. Perhaps the best way to deal with this is to remember that everyone's experience is unique and what works for one person may not work for another. This is your pregnancy and your baby, and you need to make your own decisions about what is best for you both.

HORMONAL CHANGES

The hormones in our bodies can make all the difference to how we feel and the rapidly-changing hormone levels during pregnancy inevitably play a role in your emotions. You may experience mood swings where you feel perfectly happy one moment and tearful the next; you may be irritable or forgetful. What is often described as 'pregnancy brain' may be like wading through a mental fog at times and some women feel their entire identity is changing, which may leave you wondering whether you will ever go back to 'normal'.

WORRIES ABOUT BIRTH

No one can really explain what it feels like to give birth, and no matter how much you read in advance or how many classes you go to, you can't ever know quite what will happen when your baby is ready to arrive. Worrying about giving birth, about what it will be like and about how your baby will be born is a normal part of pregnancy. You may have concerns about how much labour might hurt and how you will cope

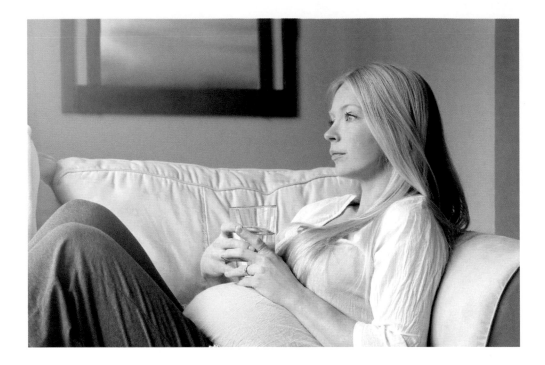

with the pain, or you may be worried about having to have interventions during labour or about losing control of what is happening and not having the birth of your choice. As you go through your pregnancy, you will have time to discuss this with your midwife or doctor and to put together a plan for the sort of birth you would like. If you have specific worries or fears, discuss these with your doctor or midwife as you are far more likely to be reassured if you take the opportunity to talk through your concerns.

Although most women have some level of anxiety about what giving birth will be like, with a minority this can become overwhelming, dominating the whole pregnancy. This is known as tokophobia (an extreme fear of giving birth). It can develop during pregnancy or may have pre-dated your pregnancy. Some women develop tokophobia if their first birth was a traumatic experience. NICE recommends that women with tokophobia should be given the opportunity to discuss their fears with a specialist healthcare professional. You should never feel embarrassed or guilty about this and discussion, relaxation therapy and counselling can all be helpful.

MENTAL HEALTH IN PREGNANCY

When we think about mental health and pregnancy and birth, there is nearly always a focus on postnatal depression as if we imagine that the time of pregnancy leading up to this will always be full of joy and feeling sad can only come after the baby is born. In fact, at least than one in ten women live with depression

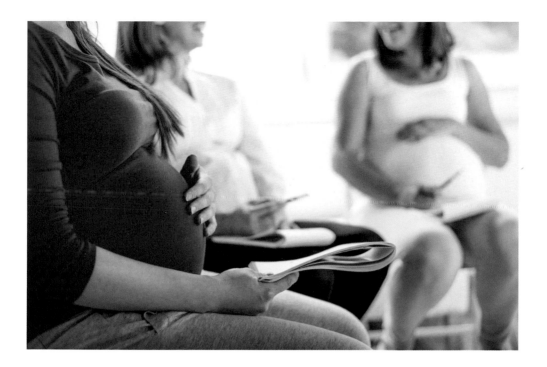

and anxiety during their pregnancy, yet antenatal depression is not always acknowledged and recognized.

Some women are at greater risk of anxiety in pregnancy, and this includes those who have had problems with mental health in the past. When you go to your antenatal appointments, you will be asked about your mental health and about any previous experience of mental health problems. All women are asked these questions, so do answer as honestly as you can because the team caring for you will be better equipped to respond to your needs if they are aware of any difficulties in the past. During pregnancy you may be very focused on your physical health and your baby's development, but your mental health is the other half of the wellbeing equation and is important too.

ANXIETY

Many women feel raised levels of anxiety during pregnancy, but if your worries are starting to mount it is worth devoting some time to looking after yourself properly and addressing your troubles rather than letting them overwhelm you:

- Talk about how you are feeling as this can help put things into perspective. Airing your anxieties can sometimes help you to realize that things are not quite as bad as you had thought. Whether you talk to your partner, to a close friend or to your midwife, telling someone about your worries can make a real difference.

- We expect a lot of ourselves as women and you may have started your pregnancy with the idea that you would waft around looking elegant in maternity clothes. The reality of feeling sick, tired and worried may leave you convinced that you are not handling pregnancy as well as you should, but you need to try to be kind to yourself. Pregnancy can be uncomfortable and exhausting. Whether it's a candlelit bath, a good book, a funny film or something else entirely that makes you feel better, allow yourself time for what you enjoy as it can help to revive your spirits.

- Sometimes when you feel anxious or worried, you may just want to curl up at home, not to see anyone and not to go out. Getting out can make all the difference to your anxiety and to how you feel about yourself, so if you can bear to drag yourself out, even briefly, you may find it is just what you need. Going for a walk or a swim or meeting up with friends may give you a boost. Sharing experiences with other women who are pregnant can also be really helpful and you may be able to meet up through pregnancy fitness or yoga classes or through antenatal groups. Even if you think groups are not your kind of thing, you may find it surprisingly helpful to spend some time with others who are at similar stages of pregnancy and to realize that you are not the only one finding things tough at times.

- When life is busy and you are feeling worried, your mind may start buzzing, leaving little space to concentrate on what is going on in the world around you. Mindfulness is a technique that aims to help you to be more aware of the present moment, to reconnect with your body and with the outside world. This can help to stop anxious thoughts dominating your mind. You can find information about mindfulness online including instruction videos, and you may want to consider going along to a mindfulness class or group to help you to learn the technique.

- Sometimes worries may make it harder to sleep at night, but getting enough sleep is important as it will help to make you feel better. Allow yourself some time to wind down properly before you go to bed, turn off your phone, iPad or laptop, try listening to a relaxation tape or having a bath and avoid eating or drinking any caffeine just before bed.

- Complementary therapies can be useful too if you are feeling stressed and anxious. Going for a massage or aromatherapy session may help, but talk to your midwife or GP to make sure they don't have any concerns and tell the therapist you are pregnant as some types of massage and some oils may not be suitable.

WHEN NOTHING SEEMS TO HELP

Sometimes you may have tried every relaxing remedy you can think of but still nothing makes a difference and your anxiety levels seem to be mounting. It can be difficult to identify exactly when feeling worried grows into something more overwhelming as this can be a gradual acceleration. There are some symptoms that suggest you should talk to your midwife or doctor about your anxiety:

- If you find it impossible to relax and you are tense, restless and on edge most of the time, feeling your worries are beyond your control
- If you have an overwhelming sense that something bad is about to happen all the time
- If you are very irritable, snappy and short-tempered
- If you can't stop dwelling on bad things that have happened in your past
- If you are constantly worried that you may have done something to upset or annoy those around you and feel you need constant reassurance
- If you feel that other people can sense your anxiety and are staring at you
- If you feel as if the world is slowing down or going faster and you are losing touch with reality
- If you have a sense of being detached from the world around you or from your own body or mind.

Sometimes anxiety can lead to physical symptoms too. You may have a panic attack in which the physical and mental symptoms of anxiety are suddenly completely overwhelming. Your heart may seem to be pounding very fast and you may be aware that you are breathing more quickly or feeling breathless. You may be sweaty, shaky or trembly, with tingling or numbness in your fingers and toes or pain in your chest. You may be weak or faint or dizzy too. If you experience this it can be frightening, but you should try to remind yourself that panic attacks do not last. Try not to fight it but to focus on slow, deep breathing. If you have ticked lots of the bullet points above or if you experience a panic attack, it is really important to discuss this with your doctor or midwife.

SUPPORT FOR MENTAL HEALTH DURING PREGNANCY

There is a growing understanding of the impact mental health problems can have during pregnancy and after giving birth. In some parts of the country there are specialist mental health services for mothers (perinatal mental health services), and you may be referred to them for support if this is needed. Sadly these services are still somewhat patchy and the provision you receive may depend entirely on where you live. Peer-to-peer support groups and local charities may be helpful if you can seek them out. It is important to get help as soon as you recognize there is a problem as this will help you to get the kind of support you need and help to prevent things becoming more serious.

CHAPTER EIGHT

Miscarriage

No one wants to think about miscarriage when they are pregnant but sadly one in four pregnancies ends in miscarriage. You may not realize quite how common it is, but the fact that it happens so often doesn't make it any less devastating if it happens to you.

One of the very frustrating things about miscarriage is that we often don't know why it has happened. The majority of women who have one or two miscarriages will go on to have a healthy baby and doctors don't usually investigate the causes of miscarriage or offer any kind of tests or treatment until women have had three miscarriages in a row. Even when tests are carried out, there may be no clear answers. This can lead women to worry that perhaps something they have or haven't done may be responsible, but most causes of miscarriage are beyond our control. Women sometimes wonder whether leading a sedentary lifestyle and wrapping themselves in cotton wool for the first few months of pregnancy might help to prevent miscarriage but there is no evidence this would have any kind of positive outcome unless doctors have advised this due to your particular circumstances. The most beneficial thing that you can do for yourself in pregnancy is to follow guidance about a healthy lifestyle with a good diet and staying active.

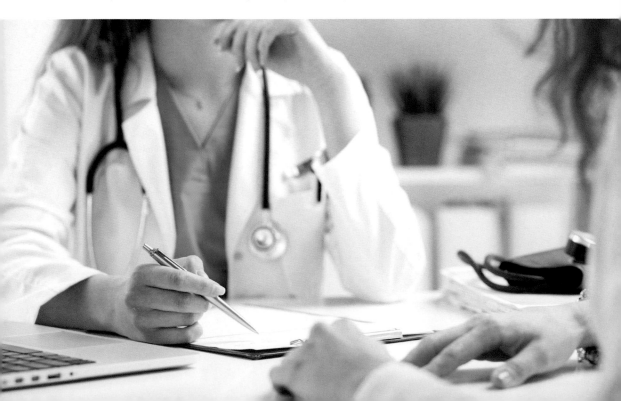

SIGNS OF MISCARRIAGE

Most miscarriages happen during the first twelve weeks of pregnancy. The thing we associate with miscarriage is bleeding in pregnancy but many women have some bleeding in perfectly healthy pregnancies. The other sign is cramping, and again it is common to have some aches and pains in early pregnancy and this may be caused by the ligaments on either side of the womb stretching. It is also possible to have a miscarriage without any signs or symptoms at all and this is known as a missed miscarriage.

If you have severe pain, persistent pain, pain on one side or any bleeding, you should always seek medical advice. Your doctor may want to do another pregnancy test to check your hormone levels or a scan. A scan is the best way of seeing what is happening inside and this may be done transvaginally (where a special ultrasound probe is inserted into your vagina) if you are in the first trimester of pregnancy. From the end of the first trimester onwards, it is most often done by putting the probe on your abdomen.

Although the majority of miscarriages happen in the first twelve weeks, later miscarriages can happen during the second trimester but this is much less common. After twenty-four weeks, pregnancy loss is referred to as a stillbirth rather than a miscarriage.

WHAT CAUSES MISCARRIAGE?

There are a number of different causes of miscarriage and some of the most common are listed below:

Chromosomal Abnormalities

Up to half of all early miscarriages are thought to happen because the embryo doesn't develop properly as a result of an abnormality in the chromosomes. This is more common in older women.

Hormonal Problems

If you have hormone problems that lead to your periods being irregular, this is often associated with fertility problems and may increase the risk of miscarriage.

Blood-Clotting Problems

Some women have antibodies in their blood that can cause clots and this can cause difficulties with the development of the placenta.

Infections

Some infections, such as listeria, chlamydia or German measles, can increase the risk of miscarriage. Things like coughs and colds are not risky, but if you have a very high fever this can lead to problems.

Changes to the Structure of the Womb

If your womb is an unusual shape or you have large fibroids (non-cancerous growths that are found in and around the womb), this may sometimes increase the risk of miscarriage.

Cervix

Sometimes the pressure of the growing baby on the cervix (neck of the womb) can make it start to open too early.

There are some existing medical conditions such as diabetes or kidney disease that can be linked to miscarriage if you are not following medical advice and taking care of yourself. This is why it is important to talk to your doctor about pre-existing medical problems and always follow their advice about how best to treat your condition when you are pregnant. The things you could do yourself that might increase your chances of losing a baby are smoking and drinking very heavily, being very overweight and taking recreational drugs while you are pregnant. Apart from this, there is very little else you could do yourself that might have an impact on either preventing a miscarriage or making it more likely to happen.

One study a while ago suggested a link between exercise and miscarriage, but when the data was analysed more closely the link was far from certain and the accepted view among most experts today is that keeping active is beneficial for you and your baby rather than harmful. Of course, it makes sense to exercise safely in pregnancy. If you have been a regular exerciser used to keeping very fit, you are unlikely to have a problem if you continue to exercise as long as you are careful about what type of exercise you do and how hard you push yourself. If you have not done any kind of exercise before, you should be more cautious but keeping active will be a positive step.

A key factor that does have an impact on your risk of having a miscarriage is your age as we know that miscarriage becomes much more common as women grow older. For a woman aged between 40 and 44, the chance of having a miscarriage is over 50 per cent and this continues to rise with age.

ECTOPIC PREGNANCY

If a fertilized egg implants in the tubes leading down from the ovaries (fallopian tubes) or anywhere else other than inside the womb, this is known as an ectopic pregnancy. An ectopic pregnancy cannot survive but you will have a positive pregnancy test. Most women experience bleeding that is not quite like a normal period (sometimes described as being dark and watery) and pain in the abdomen and sometimes the shoulders too.

If you are diagnosed with an ectopic pregnancy you may be monitored without having any further treatment as the pregnancy may stop developing naturally and the pregnancy tissue may dissolve. This monitoring is known as 'expectant management'

and is not suitable for everyone. Alternatively you may be given a drug to take to stop the pregnancy growing or you may have to have an operation to remove the ectopic which may also involve removal of the tube. The only lifestyle choice you can make that increases your risk of having an ectopic pregnancy is smoking. If you smoke there are higher levels of a protein in the fallopian tubes that can slow down the fertilized egg as it travels to the womb. Sexually transmitted infections are also linked to a higher risk of ectopic pregnancies.

EMOTIONAL SUPPORT

The emotional impact of losing a baby is often underestimated and women may worry that having lost a baby they will be more likely to experience another miscarriage. Although some women do experience recurrent miscarriage, the majority of those who have lost a baby will go on to have a healthy pregnancy.

You may think no one really understands how you feel, and other people will not always seem sympathetic. Some may avoid talking about it altogether as they do not know what to say for the best but that can feel as if they are not acknowledging your loss. You will need time and space to grieve and you need to be kind to yourself. Individuals react differently to a miscarriage, and there is no one right way to help yourself to recover. Some people find it too painful to talk about, others want to talk to friends or family and some may prefer to see a counsellor who can offer an impartial and independent listening ear. The Miscarriage Association offers information, support and advice to anyone who has been affected by miscarriage.

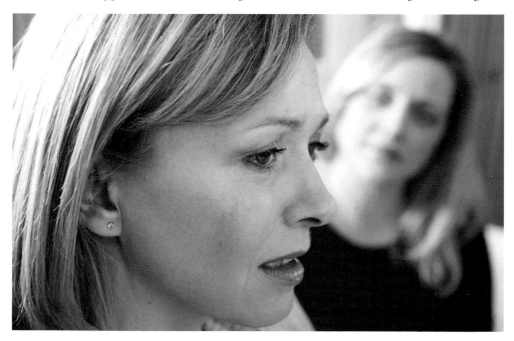

CHAPTER NINE

Common Pregnancy Health Problems

One of the things people do not always discuss about pregnancy is the range of health issues that can arise when you are expecting a baby, from bleeding gums and varicose veins to bloating and leg aches. Just looking at a list of common pregnancy health problems can feel slightly depressing as you didn't sign up for pregnancy expecting to have a selection of other health issues. The good news is that most pregnancy health problems only last for the duration of your pregnancy.

BACKACHE

Most women will find that they experience back pain at some point during pregnancy. The most common cause is the hormone called relaxin which loosens your ligaments

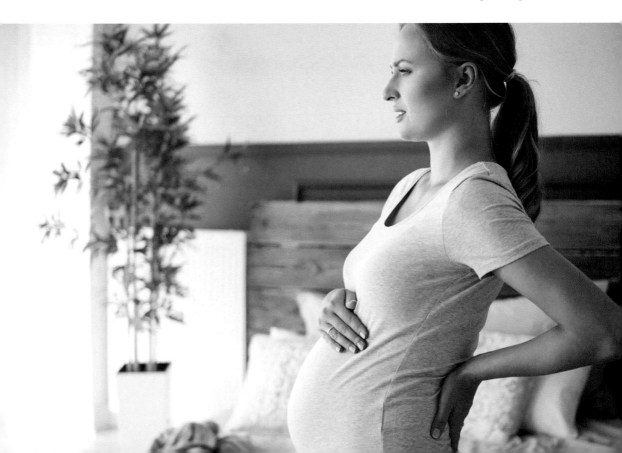

meaning that your back is carrying more of your weight than usual. This is coupled with the growing weight of your baby and an increase in progesterone which also affects your ligaments. It means that the muscles in your back may tighten up and you end up with backache.

There are some things you can do to cut your risk of getting back pain while you are pregnant. You should be careful when lifting things: avoid really heavy objects and make sure you lift properly by bending your knees to pick something up rather than bending your back. Wearing high heels can add to the pressure on your back so it is a good time to switch to flats or low heels. Make sure you get plenty of rest and try to sleep on a supportive mattress rather than a very soft one. Sleeping on your side is recommended.

Staying fit and active will help and some women find that pregnancy yoga, pregnancy Pilates, massage and swimming or antenatal aqua classes make a difference. Thinking about your posture and making sure your back is supported when you are sitting may help too. If your backache is becoming a real problem, your doctor or midwife will be able to recommend pain relief and may refer you on to an obstetric physiotherapist if they feel this is necessary.

BLEEDING GUMS

The hormonal changes of pregnancy can affect your gums which are more vulnerable to inflammation and a condition called pregnancy gingivitis, a mild form of gum disease. This can make your gums swollen and painful and they may bleed when you brush your teeth. Dental care is free for pregnant women and for a year after you have

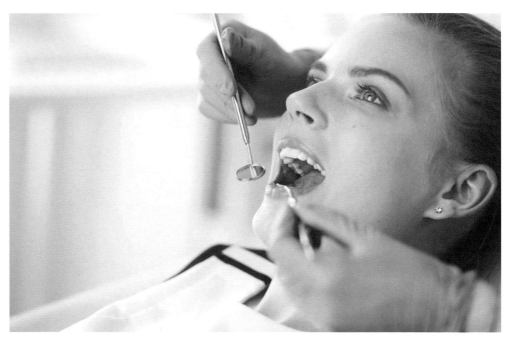

had your baby so take advantage of this and see your dentist who can give your teeth a thorough clean. Make sure your dentist knows you are pregnant as some treatments are best avoided during pregnancy.

In order to protect your gums, you need to be more careful about dental hygiene while you are pregnant. Clean your teeth twice a day with fluoride toothpaste and floss between your teeth every day. Limit your intake of sugary foods and drinks or very acidic foods (such as lemons or grapefruit) as this can help. If you are suffering with pregnancy sickness, rather than cleaning your teeth immediately after being sick, you should rinse your mouth out thoroughly with water and wait an hour or so before brushing.

BLOATING AND WIND

Bloating and wind can be a problem in pregnancy due to the increased levels of progesterone in your body which relax your muscles and slow down your digestive system. This can start in early pregnancy but may also happen later on as your baby fills up more of the space in your belly which can also affect your digestion causing more wind and bloating.

You may be able to make a difference by avoiding foods that are known to cause wind such as artichokes, beans, onions, broccoli, cabbage, leeks, sprouts and cauliflower as well as fizzy drinks. Making sure you eat slowly and chew thoroughly and sitting up properly when you eat may help. Sometimes trying to eat smaller meals throughout the day rather than two large meals at lunchtime and in the evening is a good idea. Some people swear by peppermint tea as a remedy for wind and bloating.

BLOCKED NOSE

You may notice you have a stuffy or blocked nose while you are pregnant, something known as pregnancy rhinitis. If you get it, you may also sneeze and have a runny or itchy nose. It happens because your changing hormone levels affect the mucous membranes inside your nose and it usually goes away once you have given birth. There is not a great deal you can do about it in the meantime, although you may want to see whether your local pharmacist can suggest a nasal spray which may help.

BLOOD PRESSURE

When you go for a check-up with your doctor or midwife during pregnancy they will monitor your blood pressure. It is normal for blood pressure to change a bit while you are pregnant, although you are unlikely to notice this yourself. Your blood pressure is taken by wrapping a cuff around your upper arm and inflating it to stop the blood flowing in your arm. The cuff is attached to a monitor and when it is released, the pressure of your blood can be calculated.

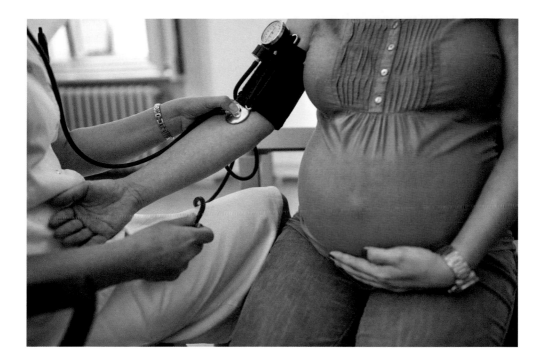

Blood pressure is measured by two figures, one on top of the other. The figure on top is called systolic blood pressure and this is the highest level of pressure as your heart pushes the blood around your body. The figure at the bottom is the diastolic blood pressure and this is the lowest pressure when your heart relaxes in between beats. During pregnancy women may experience lower than usual blood pressure in the early months and blood pressure can then rise in the second half of pregnancy. In the general population, an ideal blood pressure range is between 90/60 and 120/80, but this varies a lot in pregnancy and your midwife or doctor will tell you if they have concerns about your blood pressure.

The best things you can do yourself to keep your blood pressure healthy are to take some kind of physical exercise every day and to eat a healthy, balanced diet without too many salty foods. Do not add salt to meals either.

Some women develop high blood pressure in pregnancy, known as pregnancy-related hypertension, or others may have had high blood pressure before they became pregnant. If your blood pressure is between 140/90 and 149/99, it is classified as mild hypertension and although you will have regular checks to make sure it is stable, you are not likely to need treatment.

If your blood pressure is higher than this it may be defined as moderate (between 150/100 and 159/109) or severe (160/110 or higher) high blood pressure. You may be offered medication and if you are classified as having moderate or severe high blood pressure, you may be admitted to hospital for tests and treatment.

One of the concerns about high blood pressure in pregnancy is that it can be a sign of pre-eclampsia (see below) which affects some women, usually in the second half of pregnancy, and can be dangerous if you do not get treatment.

CARPAL TUNNEL SYNDROME

You may experience a tingling sensation or numbness in your hands and fingers during pregnancy, known as carpal tunnel syndrome. The carpal tunnel is a narrow passage that goes through the wrist and contains blood vessels, nerves and tendons. When you are pregnant, fluid can build up in the carpal tunnel and this can squash the main nerve going through your wrist. This is what causes the tingling or numbness in your hands and fingers. It happens most often during the second half of pregnancy and may be worse when you wake up in the morning. Some women find it painful and if this is the case you may want to try using an ice pack on your wrist. It will usually go once you have given birth but if it is really uncomfortable, your midwife or doctor may suggest a wrist splint.

CONSTIPATION

Many women become constipated in early pregnancy due to the hormonal changes in the body as it produces more progesterone, which relaxes muscles. When you are pregnant, this can affect the way waste products pass through your bowel as it is harder for the bowel to contract and move them along. Constipation can make you feel uncomfortable and the best way to prevent it is to ensure you are drinking plenty of water and eating lots of fruit and vegetables and high-fibre foods such as pulses and beans. Keeping active will help too. If you do get constipated, try adding wheat bran, linseed, dried prunes or apricots to your food as this may make a difference. Iron supplements can cause constipation so if your GP has prescribed them for you and they are making you constipated, ask whether there is any alternative you could be offered.

DEEP VEIN THROMBOSIS

Deep vein thrombosis or DVT happens when a blood clot develops in a vein deep inside your body, most often in your leg. You are more at risk of DVT when you are pregnant particularly if you are over 35, if you are very overweight, if you smoke and if you have a relative who has had DVT or a pulmonary embolism (see below). Women who are expecting twins or triplets are also more likely to develop DVT. Sometimes there are no symptoms when you have DVT but your leg may be swollen, tender or painful and the skin may be red and feel warm. The pain usually gets worse when you are standing or moving about.

If you think you may have DVT, see your doctor or midwife. It can be treated with injections of a drug called heparin which thins your blood and will help to dissolve the clot and make it less likely it will happen again. Having DVT and taking heparin will not have an effect on your baby.

On very rare occasions, the blood clot can get dislodged and start moving around the body in the bloodstream. If this happens and it moves to the lungs it is known as a pulmonary embolism and this can be dangerous. The symptoms include tight pain in the chest or upper back, sudden difficulty breathing and coughing up blood. If you have these symptoms, you should seek urgent medical help but pulmonary embolism is rare.

DIABETES

Sometimes women can develop a type of diabetes when they are pregnant that goes away after they have had their baby. This is known as gestational diabetes and it usually occurs in the second half of pregnancy. It can happen to anyone but is more likely if you are overweight, if you have had it in an earlier pregnancy, if you have a close relative with diabetes or have had a baby in the past that weighed more than 10lb when it was born. If your ethnic background is South Asian, Chinese, Afro-Caribbean or Middle Eastern this can also increase your likelihood of getting gestational diabetes. If you are thought to be at risk of gestational diabetes you will be offered a test for the condition.

If tests show you have gestational diabetes, you should be referred to a specialist clinic where you can learn how to deal with diabetes in pregnancy. You need to keep your blood sugar levels stable so you will be given advice about how you may be able to do this through diet and you may be prescribed medication. You will also have more check-ups during your pregnancy to make sure there are no issues as there are some additional risks for you and your baby during pregnancy, and you are more likely to have a large baby which can increase the likelihood of a Caesarean section.

DIZZINESS AND FAINTING

You may find that you feel light-headed or dizzy at times during pregnancy and pregnant women can be more prone to fainting. The most common cause is a drop in your blood pressure which can be a result of hormonal changes. It may also happen if you are dehydrated, suffering with pregnancy sickness or have low iron levels or anaemia. Talk to your GP or midwife if you have experienced fainting in pregnancy.

For dizziness, making sure that you eat properly to keep your energy levels up and drinking plenty of water will help. If you feel you are going to faint, sit down with your head between your knees or lie down and take deep breaths. It is more common to feel faint and dizzy if you are in a hot and stuffy environment so open windows or doors to let in some fresh air.

FLUID RETENTION

Your legs, ankles, feet and fingers can all swell during pregnancy because your body retains more water. The excess water may collect at the lowest parts of your body (feet and hands) and you may notice that they seem more swollen at the end of the day. This is known as oedema and it often happens in the later stages of pregnancy. If you suddenly experience fluid retention and you also have other symptoms such as a headache, visual disturbance, pain below the ribs or vomiting, this can be a sign of pre-eclampsia (see below) so you should contact your doctor or midwife.

It may sound contradictory, but drinking more water may help with fluid retention as it can flush out your body. The swelling is often worse in hot weather so avoid spending too long outside in the heat in the summer or standing for long periods, and wear comfortable shoes and socks that are not too tight.

Taking regular exercise can help to prevent swelling, and when you are sitting down try putting your feet up. Supportive pregnancy tights or leggings may be recommended. Also do not eat too many salty foods or add a lot of salt to your food.

HEADACHES

Some women find they get more headaches while they are pregnant. This is more common in the early stages of pregnancy when there are surges of hormones and the volume of blood in your body increases. Getting enough sleep and rest and drinking plenty of liquids can help to prevent headaches. If you are suffering with headaches, you may want to know whether you can take painkillers. The usual recommendation is to avoid ibuprofen or other non-steroidal anti-inflammatory drugs and any drugs containing codeine while you are pregnant. Paracetamol is the painkiller that is most often used in pregnancy, but it is always a good idea to take the lowest dose you need to make a

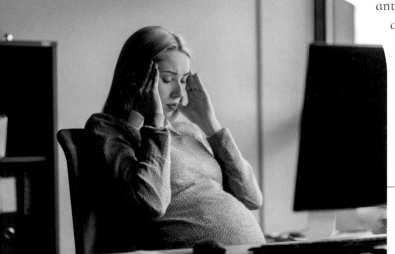

difference. If you can lie down and rest or apply a cold pack to your head that may help. Always contact your doctor or midwife if you get a very bad headache that comes on suddenly. If you have a bad headache with any sudden swelling, visual disturbance, pain below the ribs or vomiting this could be a sign of pre-eclampsia and again you should seek medical help right away.

HEARTBURN AND INDIGESTION

Heartburn and indigestion can be really uncomfortable in pregnancy. You may feel horribly full or bloated and find you can't help burping. You may have a burning feeling in your chest and a sensation of any food you have eaten coming back up your throat, leaving a bitter taste at the back of your mouth. You may be sick or feel sick. If heartburn and indigestion are so bad that they are stopping you eating properly and you are losing weight or having stomach pains, see your doctor or midwife about this.

Heartburn and indigestion are caused by changes in your body and by your growing baby pressing on your stomach, so eating more smaller meals throughout the day can be beneficial rather than large meals at lunchtime and in the evening. Avoiding spicy, fried or fatty foods may help too. Alcohol and smoking can both cause indigestion and are best avoided in pregnancy for other health reasons. Some women find that drinking milk or eating yoghurt can help.

LEG ACHE AND CRAMPS

Pregnant women are prone to leg cramps where the muscles in your legs suddenly become tight and painful. It often happens at night. Stretching the muscle by straightening and flexing your leg and foot and massaging the muscle may help. It is not entirely clear why leg cramps are more common in pregnancy but keeping active during the day, doing some stretching exercises and drinking plenty of water may help to reduce your risk of cramps.

NAUSEA AND SICKNESS

Unfortunately the majority of women experience some degree of nausea and sickness during pregnancy. You may just feel nauseous rather than actually being sick, but around seven out of every ten women have what is often known as pregnancy sickness or morning sickness, although it can occur at any time of the day. Pregnancy sickness is thought to be caused by hormonal changes and is apparently more common in first pregnancies and in women who suffer from motion sickness and who get migraines. You are more likely to experience morning sickness if you are expecting twins or triplets. It can make early pregnancy feel a bit grim, but for the majority of women it will gradually disappear as the pregnancy progresses.

There are some things you can do to make a difference. Dry toast or plain crackers can be tolerable if you feel nauseous, and eating more regular smaller meals can help. Women often find that the smell of cooking and of certain foods is off-putting so plain food such as bread, rice or pasta may be preferable. Ginger is sometimes suggested as a cure for pregnancy sickness, so you can see whether ginger tea or ginger biscuits help you.

As previously mentioned, some women suffer a severe form of morning sickness known as hyperemesis gravidarum when they can't keep any food down at all. If you experience this you may need to take medication or be given treatment in hospital if you are dehydrated.

NOSEBLEEDS

They may not be a pregnancy symptom you have anticipated, but around 20 per cent of women have a nosebleed when they are expecting a baby. As with many other pregnancy-related problems, nosebleeds in pregnancy are caused by your changing hormones which can make small blood vessels in your nose expand and this can lead them to burst. If you've never had a nosebleed before it can be a bit alarming, but you need to sit down leaning forwards and either pinch your nose or put an ice pack on the bridge of your nose. There is usually nothing to worry about with a nosebleed, but if the bleeding won't stop, seek medical advice.

PELVIC PAIN

As many as one in five pregnant women experience pelvic pain but it can feel different for different women, so it may just be an aching in the pelvic area or may be more severe pain felt around the groin, pelvis or even lower back and abdomen. You may experience a clicking or grinding feeling in the pelvic area and it is often worse when you are physically active. This kind of pain is known as Pregnancy-related Pelvic Girdle Pain. For some women, it can be really debilitating if walking becomes painful and it starts to affect your sleep. If you are suffering with Pregnancy-related Pelvic Girdle Pain, you may be referred to a physiotherapist who can help with exercises to restore normal movement and to strengthen the muscles in your pelvic area.

If you are experiencing persistent severe pain, or it is regularly coming and going and is associated with other symptoms such as nausea and vomiting, your waters breaking or your baby moving less frequently, you should seek medical advice right away.

PILES

Sometimes during pregnancy the blood vessels around your bottom can swell causing haemorrhoids, also known as piles. They can be inside or outside your bottom, and sometimes people don't even realize they have them. They are more common in pregnancy for a number of reasons: the hormonal changes in your body, the pressure of your growing womb on the veins underneath and constipation. Piles can cause bleeding from your bottom and may be itchy or achey. It may be uncomfortable when you have a poo and the piles may sometimes stick out from your bottom.

One of the most important things you can do if you have haemorrhoids is to make sure you don't get constipated as this can make them worse. Drink lots of water, and have plenty of fruit and vegetables. Dried fruit such as apricots or prunes may help if you are constipated. There are creams you can buy at the chemist to help ease the symptoms, but check that anything you use is suitable for pregnancy. If they are really uncomfortable and causing you problems, your midwife or doctor may be able to offer further advice.

PRE-ECLAMPSIA

This condition is most common in the later stages of pregnancy, usually after the twentieth week. Having high blood pressure is a sign of pre-eclampsia, along with protein in your urine. You may also experience headaches and vision problems, swollen feet or hands, dizziness and pain below the ribs.

Pre-eclampsia only occurs in around 6 per cent of pregnancies and you may be slightly more at risk if you are carrying twins or triplets, if you are over 40, if you are very overweight, if you have diabetes, high blood pressure or kidney disease. You are also at higher risk if you have a family history of pre-eclampsia, or if you have had it yourself in an earlier pregnancy, if it is more than ten years since you had your last baby, if you have lupus (an autoimmune disease) or if you have antiphospholipid syndrome (a condition that causes an increased risk of blood clots).

If you are diagnosed with pre-eclampsia you may be admitted to hospital until your baby is born where you will usually be given medication to lower your blood pressure. The only way to completely cure pre-eclampsia is to give birth, so you may need to be induced or have a Caesarean section. There are some conditions that can develop if you have pre-eclampsia and they may affect your liver, blood or organs. There is also a risk of eclampsia, a very rare condition that causes fits and can be life-threatening.

RESTLESS LEGS

If you feel an irresistible urge to move your legs around after sitting for a while or when you are in bed, you may be suffering from a condition known as Restless Legs Syndrome which can affect women during pregnancy. Restless Legs Syndrome is sometimes described as tingly, itchy, tickly, buzzy, burning or just plain uncomfortable and you may have an overwhelming need to move your legs to relieve the sensation.

It most often happens when you are in bed or after you have been sitting still for a long time, and moving your legs about can make it feel better. Massage, warm baths, stretching and relaxation techniques may all help to relieve the symptoms. The good news is that it usually goes away soon after having your baby.

SLEEPLESSNESS

Sleep can be disturbed in pregnancy if you find you need to get up during the night to pee, if you have restless legs syndrome or if you have difficulty finding a comfortable position in bed. Some women have strange dreams or nightmares when they are pregnant and this can affect your quality of sleep too, as can any worries or anxieties you have about your pregnancy. It is important to get as much rest as you can, but try not to stress about lack of sleep as it won't affect your baby.

If you are having problems sleeping, the general advice for anyone suffering from insomnia may help, so no caffeine in the afternoon and evening, don't eat too close to going to bed and no TV, laptops, tablets or mobile phones in the bedroom or in the hour or so before you try to go to sleep. Some find that a warm bath and a milky drink helps too. Lying in bed worrying about not sleeping can make it even harder to drop off and if you are finding it impossible to get to sleep, it is sometimes better to read for a while and then try again.

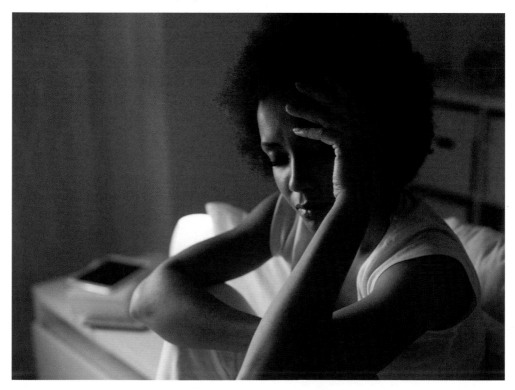

HOW TO STAY FIT AND HEALTHY DURING PREGNANCY

STRESS INCONTINENCE OR URINARY PROBLEMS

Most pregnant women need to pee more than usual. In early pregnancy this is largely down to hormonal changes but as pregnancy advances, the weight of the baby pressing down on your bladder is usually to blame. If you find you are waking up in the night needing to pee, try not to drink too much just before going to bed.

For many pregnant women, it is not just needing to pee more frequently that is an issue but also releasing urine involuntarily. This can happen if you sneeze or cough, or if you do certain types of exercise. If you are experiencing what is known as stress incontinence, you must do your pelvic floor exercises to strengthen your pelvic floor and you need to carry on doing them after the birth too. If pregnancy-related incontinence is an issue, talk to your midwife.

If you are peeing a lot and it stings, if you find it hard to produce much urine or your urine is cloudy, you may have a urinary tract infection which is more common in pregnancy. A urine test can tell whether or not you have an infection and it is easily treated with antibiotics. Cranberry juice is often recommended for urinary infections, although there is no scientific evidence that it helps.

SWOLLEN FEET

Your feet and ankles can swell up during pregnancy and this is usually a result of fluid retention (see above). It can also be a sign of pre-eclampsia, so ask your doctor or midwife about it.

STRETCH MARKS

The majority of women (around 80 per cent) get stretch marks during pregnancy which are caused by the skin stretching to accommodate your growing bump. They are most often found on your abdomen where they appear as pink or purple indented streaks, but you may also get them on your breasts or thighs and they can feel itchy. The good news is that they will gradually fade after pregnancy, although you will be left with fine pale lines. There are lots of different creams and oils you can buy that claim they can prevent stretch marks or cause them to fade, but in reality whether you get stretch marks or not depends on the elasticity of your skin.

TENDER BREASTS

One of the first signs that you are pregnant can be tender breasts and your breasts and nipples may feel very sensitive. Your breasts are likely to swell during pregnancy as they prepare for breastfeeding and they may feel uncomfortable and heavy or even painful. You may notice that the veins on your breasts become more noticeable too.

Make sure you have a well-fitted, supportive and comfortable bra. There are some specialist shops where they will measure you properly for a bra, but bear in mind that you may change size more than once during your pregnancy.

TIREDNESS

This is often one of the first symptoms of pregnancy and for some women it feels more like complete and utter exhaustion than tiredness. The huge changes your body is going through are usually responsible and rest is really the only cure. Take any opportunity you can to go to bed early or to rest at other times of the day if you are very weary, and make sure you are eating properly and drinking enough liquids. Most women find that their energy returns once they are through the first trimester of pregnancy, but you may start feeling tired again as you approach the final months of pregnancy. Sometimes if you are feeling very tired in pregnancy this can be due to low levels of iron (anaemia). Iron levels are analysed when you have a blood test at your pregnancy check-up and you may be prescribed some kind of supplement if your levels are low. If you have any concerns about this, discuss it with your midwife.

VAGINAL BLEEDING

If you have vaginal bleeding at any stage of pregnancy you may worry that you are losing your baby, but in fact many women who go on to have perfectly healthy babies have some bleeding during pregnancy. In the very early stages of pregnancy, you may

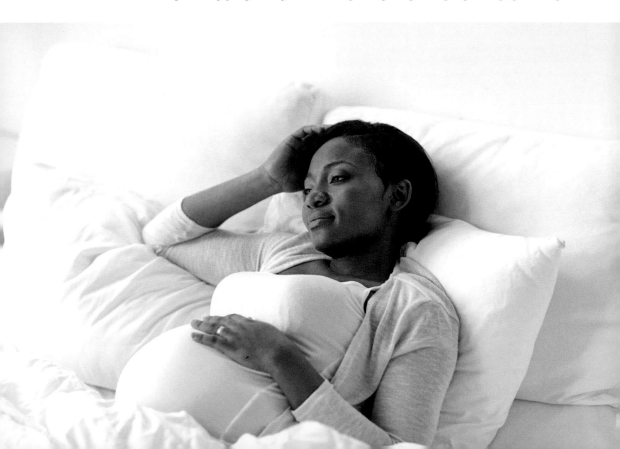

experience what is known as implantation bleeding which happens when the embryo implants into the soft lining of the womb. Changes to the cervix, or neck of the womb, can also cause bleeding in pregnancy. Although light spotting is not uncommon, talk to your doctor or midwife about any kind of bleeding when you are pregnant.

In later pregnancy there are a number of conditions that can cause bleeding, mainly to do with the placenta which may be lying low in the womb or may be coming away from the wall of the womb. Vaginal bleeding can also signal miscarriage and you should always seek medical advice about this.

VAGINAL DISCHARGE

Most women find they have more vaginal discharge than usual during pregnancy. This is usually clear or white in colour and there is no cause for concern unless it is itchy and changes colour (becoming more yellow or greenish). This could indicate a vaginal infection so see your doctor if you are experiencing these signs. There is often an increase in discharge towards the end of pregnancy too. If you have a lot of watery discharge you should get medical advice as there is a chance your waters may have broken.

VARICOSE VEINS

The increased blood flow in pregnancy can cause your veins to swell, and this along with the pressure of your growing womb can lead to the veins becoming enlarged. This most often happens to the veins in your legs and they may look lumpy and a blue or purple colour, but some women also get varicose veins around the entrance to the vagina. Varicose veins are not harmful but they can feel uncomfortable.

There are things you can do to help prevent varicose veins, but you are more likely to get them if other members of your family have had them. Standing or sitting still for long periods of time can make them worse, so try to move around when you can. If you are at a desk all day, don't sit with your legs crossed and try to exercise your legs at your desk by circling your feet around in both directions or by bending your feet backwards and forwards. Keeping your feet raised is recommended too. You can buy special support (or compression) tights and leggings which may help. Putting on weight can cause varicose veins and pregnancy inevitably involves getting heavier, but being active and making sure you eat healthily will ensure you don't gain too much too quickly. Usually varicose veins will improve after you have given birth.

CHAPTER TEN

Complementary Therapies

Whether it's an aromatherapy massage or some herbal supplements, complementary therapies have become much more mainstream in the last couple of decades and there is a growing interest in what are often seen as more natural and holistic treatments for a range of issues. However, once you are pregnant you need to exercise more caution about complementary therapies as there may not be robust evidence about their safety for pregnant women and so discussing anything you intend to try with your midwife or doctor is always advisable. NICE says that few complementary therapies have been established as being safe and effective in pregnancy and suggests 'Women should not assume that such therapies are safe and they should be used as little as possible during pregnancy.'

Perhaps the biggest risks are assuming that a therapy that is labelled 'natural' is inevitably safe or substituting complementary therapies for prescribed conventional medicines. You should also use caution when mixing complementary therapies with traditional medicines as there may be interactions that can impact on the effectiveness of the medicine.

If you are going to see a complementary therapist, make sure that your therapist knows you are pregnant, and that they are registered with an appropriate body to show they are properly qualified.

Some midwives may have additional training in complementary therapies to offer treatments such as massage, aromatherapy, reflexology and acupuncture, although the Royal College of Midwives makes it clear that complementary and natural remedies should be used 'in conjunction with conventional midwifery and obstetric care, and not viewed by mothers or midwives as a replacement for adequate monitoring and care by appropriately qualified maternity professionals.'

ACUPUNCTURE

This is a traditional Chinese form of treatment that involves sticking very fine needles into the skin at specific points along what are believed to be the body's energy lines. It is thought your life force, or Qi, travels along these energy lines, known as meridians. If there are blockages and the Qi can't move freely, this is believed to cause health problems. The needles used in acupuncture aim to help stimulate the Qi so it can flow

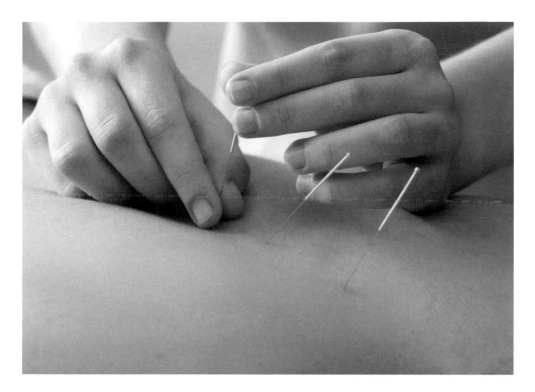

around the meridians. If you go for an acupuncture session, the acupuncturist will check how the Qi is flowing in your body which they do by feeling the pulses on your wrists and looking at your tongue as the colour and coating of your tongue gives them a view of your overall health.

Acupuncture also aims to restore the balance in the body. In traditional Chinese belief, everything is divided into Ying and Yang, which are like two sides of the same coin. Everything in nature is believed to be a balance of these two opposite forces. In your body, one of these may dominate; you may have too much or too little of either or both. Acupuncture aims to help restore the balance so your body can be in harmony and balanced, with Ying and Yang proportionate to one another and blended together into a whole.

Acupuncture may be recommended in pregnancy if you are experiencing back pain or pelvic pain. It is also used for a variety of other pregnancy issues such as headaches, tiredness and morning sickness. There is some research evidence to suggest acupuncture may be effective in treating back and pelvic pain in pregnancy. It is sometimes used to try to bring on labour and there is some limited evidence that it may help to prepare the cervix, or neck of the womb, for giving birth. Women who have used acupuncture previously may decide to have acupuncture for pain relief in labour and there is some evidence that this may be effective, but you need to ensure your acupuncturist has experience of working with women who are giving birth.

Acupressure

This could be described as acupuncture without the needles, as acupressure uses the same theory of meridians that channel energy but rather than using a needle, pressure is applied to specific points in the body with fingers and thumbs instead. The idea is that this will allow the energy to flow freely through the body by clearing any blockages.

One common use of acupressure in pregnancy is to help with morning sickness. You can buy acupressure wristbands with a little button that applies pressure to the point on the wrist said to be responsible for morning sickness. Some women feel they help, and although there is no clear scientific evidence that they can reduce sickness, they are unlikely to do any harm either.

Acupressure may also be recommended for pain relief in labour and there is some evidence that it may be helpful, although more research is needed.

ALEXANDER TECHNIQUE

A technique focused on posture, the Alexander Technique is based on the idea that the way you sit, stand and move can affect your physical health. The Alexander Technique focuses on increasing self-awareness not just about posture, where you are encouraged to sit and stand properly rather than slouching, but also in terms of how you think about yourself, a bit like mindfulness, so it can also help with stress and anxiety. You can learn the Alexander Technique in classes or one-to-one lessons. It is said to be particularly helpful for problems such as back pain, neck pain, muscle tension and stiffness and poor posture. There is some evidence it has a positive outcome on back and neck pain, and it may be recommended if you are experiencing pain in pregnancy.

AROMATHERAPY

Although there is no solid scientific evidence aromatherapy has a role to play in curing disease or illness, it can be very calming and many people use aromatic essential oils to help with relaxation and improve their overall sense of wellbeing. The oils, which come from plants, seeds and flowers, can be used for an aromatherapy massage, diffused into the air in an oil burner or a few drops can be added to bath water.

While you are pregnant, you need to be more cautious about aromatherapy as there are some oils that should not be used in pregnancy. Working out which oils are safe to use during pregnancy is not straightforward as views seem to differ on the oils that may be risky for women who are expecting. If you have any existing medical conditions or are taking any medication, you should be particularly careful. It is always a good idea to check with your midwife or doctor before using essential oils, and if you go for an aromatherapy session, make sure the therapist knows that you are pregnant.

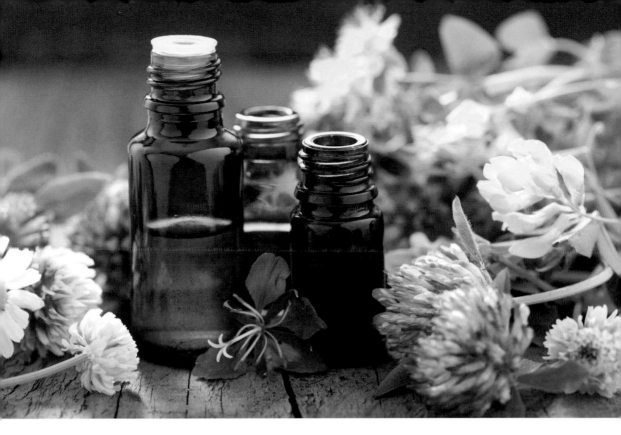

Generally women are advised not to use essential oils for massage during the first trimester of pregnancy, and they should also be avoided if you have thyroid problems, high or low blood pressure or diabetes. Be careful if buying essential oils yourself as cheaper oils may be mixed with a variety of substances to dilute them so they should be used with caution.

Bach Flower Remedies

Named after Dr Edward Bach who first started using them in the early 1900s, these are remedies made from wild flowers soaked or boiled with water and mixed with brandy, although you can also buy alcohol-free Bach Flower Remedies. There are thirty-eight different remedies used to help with different conditions and each one is associated with a different emotion or characteristic. Dr Bach saw the physical illness as an outward sign of an emotional difficulty, so to work out which remedy you need you have to try to work out the emotional state behind the physical nature of any problem you have by concentrating on how it makes you feel emotionally. The remedies are mixed together to get the right combination for your individual situation and you add drops of the different remedies to water which you drink. Perhaps the best-known Bach Flower Remedy is Rescue Remedy which is meant to help people to deal with a crisis or emergency. It is a blend of Rock Rose, Impatiens, Cherry Plum, Star of Bethlehem and Clematis, and was created by Dr Bach himself.

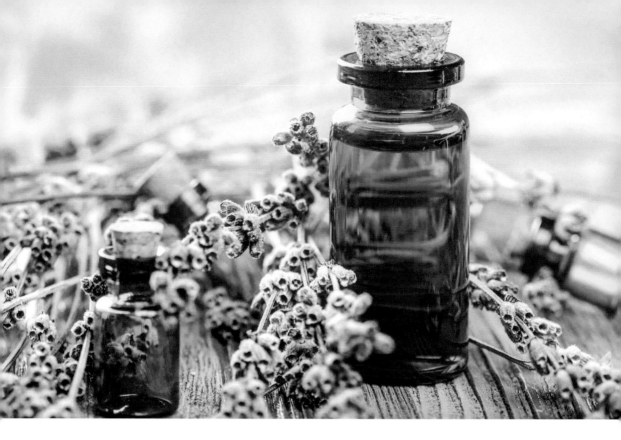

Bach Flower Remedies are not generally considered to be unsafe but, as with any complementary therapy, it is always a good idea to discuss using them with your midwife or doctor.

CHIROPRACTIC

This therapy treats problems of the bones, muscles, nerves and joints and looks at the effect these can have on a person's nervous system and overall health and wellbeing. A chiropractor uses manipulation (which they may refer to as adjustments) to try to restore normal function to the body. It is most often known as a treatment for backache and may be used for this in pregnancy.

HERBAL MEDICINE

There is sometimes an idea that any herbal medicine must be safer than conventional medicine because it is 'natural', but in fact you should be just as careful, if not more so, with herbal remedies. Some herbal remedies may not be safe for use in pregnancy, and herbal medicines are not always standardized so a medicine may be of very different strengths depending on which one you buy. The quality may also differ from one brand to another. There are not the same strict regulations about quality or the level of active ingredients for herbal medicines as there are with conventional medicine.

It is always advisable to go to a qualified practitioner and to check with a medical professional about any herbal medicine you are considering taking in pregnancy.

HOMEOPATHY

The theory behind homeopathic treatment is that 'like cures like' and so it uses tiny quantities of substances that can produce the symptoms of an illness in order to treat the illness itself. The substances used are very diluted and practitioners believe the more the remedy is diluted, the more potent it becomes as it loses any impurities. Homeopathic remedies are often given as a pill but may also be offered as an ointment, powder or solution. You will find homeopathic remedies for a range of pregnancy problems such as morning sickness and nausea, constipation, backache and heartburn. Although you can buy remedies in a local health food store, it is recommended that you see a qualified homeopath rather than purchasing remedies over the counter as they will be able to tailor the remedy to you and will offer holistic treatment rather than focusing on one single ailment.

Homeopathy is sometimes used to try to bring on labour and there have been a few trials to look at the evidence into this, but more research is needed before it can be proven to be effective. There is also a range of homeopathic remedies that may be recommended during labour and you may even find homeopathic birth kits, containing a selection of remedies and instructions for their use.

Homeopathy is a widely-used and popular complementary treatment and was even offered in some NHS settings, but in 2010 the House of Commons Science and Technology Committee concluded that the scientific basis for the idea of like-for-like

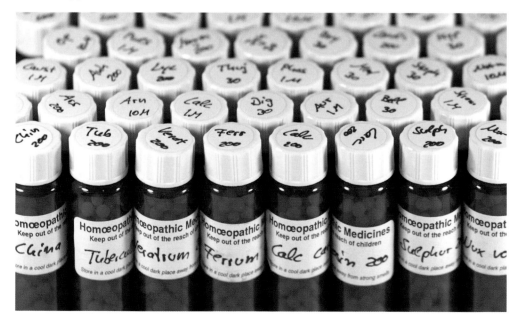

cures was 'theoretically weak' and the idea that homeopathic dilutions carried an imprint of the substances dissolved in them was 'scientifically implausible'. They recognized some patients found homeopathy to be effective but concluded this was most likely due to the placebo effect.

HYPNOTHERAPY

Our views of hypnotherapy are often coloured by stage hypnotherapists who hypnotize members of their audience on stage to get them to act in ways they would never normally consider, so perhaps the first and most important thing to stress about hypnotherapy is that hypnosis only works if you are willing to be hypnotized. A hypnotherapist uses hypnosis to take you, if you are willing to be taken there, into a relaxed trance-like state that is similar to the way you might feel when you are daydreaming. The aim of this is to allow them to work with your subconscious to relieve any fears or anxieties that may lie beneath the surface. A hypnotherapist can also teach you the basics of self-hypnosis which you can use to help yourself feel more calm and relaxed when you are at home.

Hypnotherapy may be used in labour as a form of pain relief and you may also come across what is known as hypnobirthing. This is not hypnotherapy but uses visualization and mindfulness techniques to help you to relax in labour and it is often taught in classes. Although there is no clear scientific evidence to prove it works as a form of pain relief, some women find it helps to reduce anxiety and stress.

MASSAGE

We know massage can be relaxing and there is some evidence it may help with anxiety and insomnia in pregnancy. It may also be used to help with backache and to relieve pain in labour. There are some concerns about massage in the first three

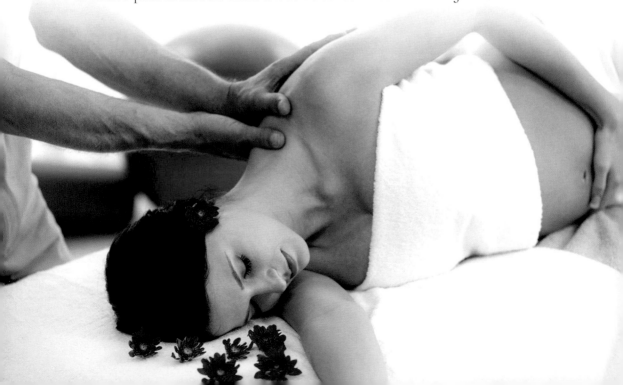

months of pregnancy, so it is best to avoid abdominal massage at this time. You should always make sure that anyone giving you a massage knows that you are expecting a baby.

MOXIBUSTION

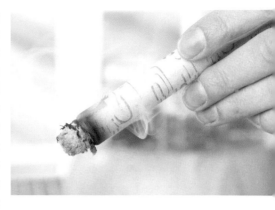

This is a traditional Chinese medicine which may be suggested if you have a breech baby, with their feet or bottom down, and you want to try to help it to turn so the head is facing down instead to be ready for birth. Moxibustion uses a dried herb called moxa or mugwort which is tightly compacted into what looks like a large cigar. One end of the cigar is lit and once it is smouldering, it is held over the side of the smallest toe on each foot for about fifteen minutes every day for up to a fortnight. There is some evidence moxibustion may have a role to play in turning breech babies; it is thought it could help to release hormones that stimulate the muscles of the womb which in turn encourages the baby to turn.

REFLEXOLOGY

Although we usually think of reflexology as foot massage, it may involve other parts of your body such as your lower legs, hands, face or ears. The theory behind reflexology is similar to the idea of acupuncture: that certain places on your feet and these other areas, known as reflex points, correspond to specific organs in your body. The reflexologist applies gentle pressure to these reflex points to try to restore your body's natural balance.

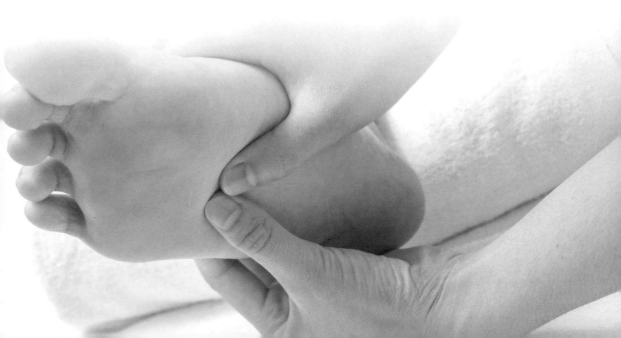

Reflexology is not considered risky during pregnancy but, as with any complementary therapy, discuss it with your midwife and make sure you are seeing a qualified reflexologist. Some reflexologists prefer not to treat women during the first trimester of pregnancy. Before the session begins, the reflexologist will spend time asking questions about your medical history and your pregnancy. They will then apply pressure to some of your reflex points; this aims to stimulate the flow of energy in your body and help it to repair any problems.

Although different forms of reflexology foot massage have been used for centuries, the mapping of reflex points used today was not drawn up until the 1900s but it has become a popular therapy in recent years. Many people find reflexology very relaxing and it may help to relieve anxiety and tension and thus improve your sense of wellbeing. During pregnancy it is often used to help with sleep problems and anxiety and with tiredness too.

SHIATSU

The word Shiatsu means 'finger pressure' in Japanese and this is a massage technique based on traditional theories of Oriental medicine. A Shiatsu practitioner will not just use their fingers but may also use their thumbs, palms, elbows and even knees to apply pressure to points in the body with the aim of ensuring that energy, or the life force, runs freely through the body. You may be relieved to learn it is a type of massage that doesn't involve taking your clothes off. Shiatsu practitioners aim not just to even out energy imbalances in the body, but also to reduce tension in the muscles and ease stiff joints in order to relax the body. Shiatsu may be recommended for any aches and pains you experience during pregnancy or to help with any stress or tension you are feeling by helping

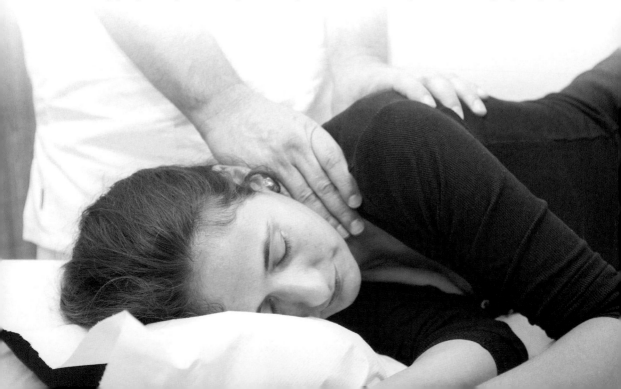

you to relax, which may also improve your overall sense of wellbeing. Some Shiatsu practitioners specialize in women's health and maternity, and it can also be used in labour to help with pain relief.

SO SHOULD I USE COMPLEMENTARY THERAPIES IN PREGNANCY?

It is clear that many women find complementary therapies helpful during pregnancy and labour, and some midwives may offer these therapies too. Although there is not a great deal of scientific evidence to prove that many of them are effective, this does not mean individual women do not find them helpful.

There are some key points to consider with any alternative form of therapy in pregnancy.

- Always use a therapist who is a registered practitioner or member of the regulatory body of whichever therapy you intend to use
- Tell the therapist you are pregnant before any treatment starts
- Make sure they are also aware of any other medical conditions you may have or any medication you are taking
- Check with your doctor or midwife about any therapy you intend to use
- Don't assume that natural means safe; use the same caution that you would with taking any other medicine before using any complementary therapy in pregnancy.

CHAPTER ELEVEN

Preparing for Birth

The idea of giving birth may seem far away if you can barely see your bump, but your midwife may start talking about what sort of birth you want far earlier in pregnancy than you might have anticipated. You may have definite thoughts about the sort of birth you want from the start if you know you would like a home birth or if you definitely want to have your baby in hospital, but many women don't begin their pregnancy with particularly fixed views and you may feel uncertain about choosing where would be the best place for you to have your baby or how would be the best way to do it. The most important thing to bear in mind is that what is right for someone else is not necessarily right for you and what other people say or think may not be relevant to you. There can be a sense that certain ways of giving birth are somehow 'better' than others, but the only type of birth that is better is what is right for you and your baby.

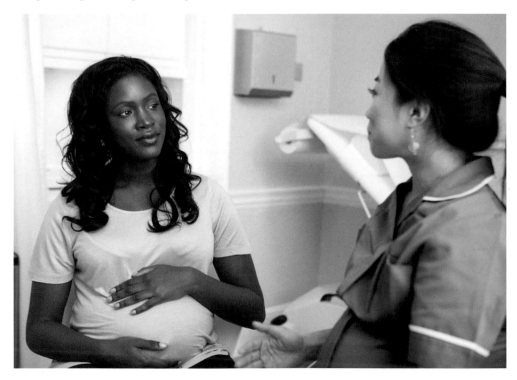

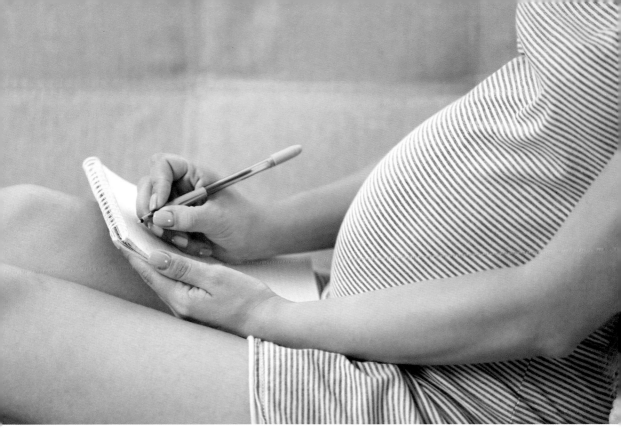

BIRTH PLAN

Your midwife will talk to you about your thoughts regarding birth and you will be encouraged to write a birth plan. This is an opportunity to think about your baby's birth and ask any questions you may have and to discuss your preferences, taking your individual circumstances into account. You will not just want to think about where you would like to give birth but also what kind of pain relief you would like, who you would like with you when you have your baby, whether you would like any special facilities such as a birthing pool, etc. No matter what you decide in advance, things may not go according to plan when your baby is born so you need to allow for some flexibility. Although it is possible to give quite a lot of detail about the sort of birth you would like in your birth plan, it is best to think of the plan as a guide rather than a set of rules you have laid down for yourself.

PAIN RELIEF IN LABOUR

Women are often worried about how they will cope with pain in labour but there is a range of different types of pain relief you may want to consider, from simple breathing exercises to anaesthetics that block pain. Finding out about all the different options will enable you to make an informed decision about this and to help you to think about what you would like to say about pain relief in your birth plan. This is not set in stone and you can change your mind about pain relief when you are in labour; in England around a quarter of women do change their minds about this when they are giving birth.

Every woman's experience of labour and the pain of labour is different, but a contraction is often described as being like a strong period pain which feels worse as the muscles of the womb tighten up and then gradually subsides. Being fit and healthy during your pregnancy does help when it comes to labour and one recent study found that women who did aerobic exercise during pregnancy tended to have a shorter labour time. It is also useful to be informed about the stages of labour and to know what to expect as this may help to reduce your anxiety about labour pain.

Many women find that simple breathing exercises can help, particularly in the early stages of labour, and these are often taught in pregnancy yoga classes. If yoga isn't for you, you can find information about this online. Some women like to listen to music, use ice packs or choose to have a bath or shower or move about to help ease early labour pain. You may decide to use a birthing ball, which looks like the large round balls you get at the gym, as this can help with pain relief in labour but it's a good idea to have tried it out during pregnancy to get used to it.

You may choose to use complementary therapies which can help you to feel more relaxed and some midwives may use therapies such as aromatherapy or massage. Other commonly-used therapies for labour pain include acupuncture, homeopathy, hypnosis, massage and reflexology. There is limited scientific evidence about the impact these may have on labour pain, but some research has shown that

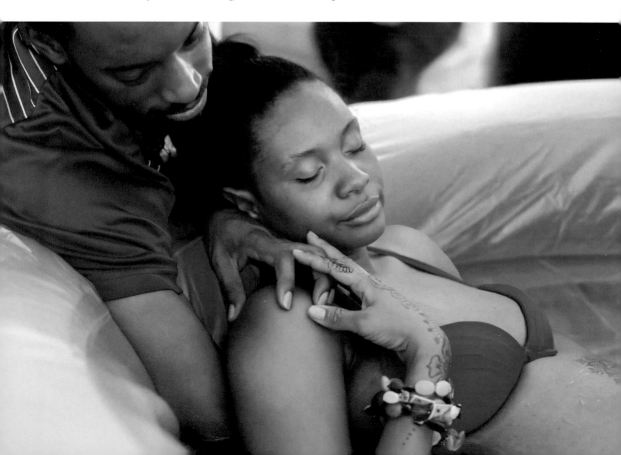

acupuncture and self-hypnosis could make a difference. There are also classes that teach hypnobirthing and you can find some free resources for this online.

Having a birthing pool can also help with pain relief and this has become an increasingly popular choice. If you are having your baby at home you can hire a pool, and birthing centres or midwife-led units often have birthing pools as do some hospitals. You don't have to actually give birth in the pool if you are using one as you can use it for pain relief in labour and get out when it is time to push your baby out.

A TENS (transcutaneous electrical nerve stimulation) machine may sound slightly alarming, but it uses electrical impulses to dull pain through sticky pads on leads that are attached to your skin. TENS machines are used for pain relief for problems such as arthritis or back pain and can be used in labour. TENS is not painful but gives you a tingling feeling from the electrical impulses. You can hire a TENS machine from a pharmacy if you want to use one in labour.

The most common form of pain relief is gas and air, or nitrous oxide, and around three-quarters of women use it during labour. Nitrous oxide is usually available wherever you choose to have your baby as midwives can carry it with them for home births. It can make you feel a bit woozy or light-headed but it doesn't have any impact on your baby.

A pain-killing injection of pethidine is another option but this is not recommended for the final stages of labour as it takes a while to work and lasts for a few hours. Some women don't like the way it makes them feel and it passes through the placenta to your baby, making them drowsy or sometimes affecting their breathing.

An epidural is used by close to a third of women in labour and this is an anaesthetic that is injected into your back and aims to block pain. It does not pass through the placenta to the baby and is a very effective method of pain relief for many women but it doesn't always work for everyone. It can only be given by an anaesthetist so you can only have an epidural if you have your baby in hospital. It can make the second stage of labour longer as women don't always know when they need to push if they've had an epidural.

WHERE TO HAVE YOUR BABY

Women are not always aware that they should have a choice of where they give birth. You should be able to decide to have your baby in hospital, in a unit run by midwives or at home, although what is recommended for you may depend on your individual circumstances. If you have had difficulties in pregnancy or have certain medical issues, this will affect your choices about where to have your baby.

Hospital Birth
Most women in the UK have their babies in a maternity unit in hospital. If you choose to do this, the main advantage is that you have access to all the services a hospital can offer. There will be specialist doctors who can help if your birth becomes complicated,

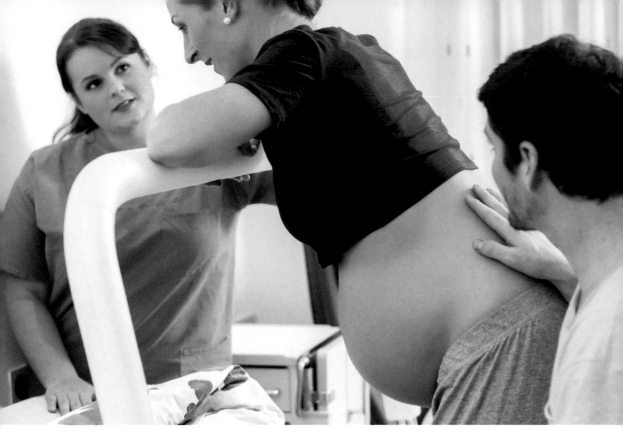

if you need pain relief and if your baby needs any special care after they are born. If you choose to have your baby in hospital, it may not be possible to be looked after by a midwife you know already, and you are more likely to have medical intervention such as forceps or a ventouse (a vacuum device that uses suction) to help with the birth.

Midwifery Unit

There are two types of units led by midwives. Some midwife-led units are attached to hospitals which makes it very easy to move you to be cared for by an obstetrician during labour if this becomes necessary. Others are freestanding units and are not part of a hospital. Midwife-led units are sometimes referred to as birth centres. These units usually feel more friendly and relaxed than a hospital ward and there is likely to be a birthing pool. There is a greater chance of being looked after by a midwife you have met during your pregnancy at a midwife-led unit and you are less likely to have any intervention, but you will not have access to an epidural.

Home Birth

Although we hear a lot about home birth, across England and Wales only about 2 per cent of women have their babies at home. Choosing a home birth gives you the opportunity to have your baby in familiar surroundings which may be more relaxing, with whoever you wish to be present and where you are less likely to have

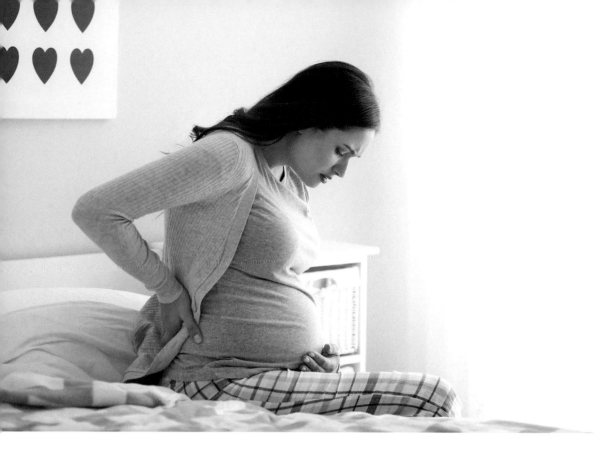

interventions. Giving birth at home does mean that you would not have access to the full range of pain relief available in hospital, such as an epidural. There is always a possibility that you may need to transfer to hospital, particularly if this is your first baby, and you should bear this in mind. One large study found that 45 per cent of women having a first baby and 12 per cent of women having another baby transferred to hospital when they had planned for a home birth.

There is also a small increase in risk of problems for women who have their first baby at home; the results of the same study found that there were about 9.3 adverse outcomes for every 1,000 planned home births compared with about 5.3 for every 1,000 births planned in obstetric units in hospitals. This does not apply to women who have already had a baby, where home birth outcomes are generally similar or slightly better.

WAITING FOR YOUR BABY

Apparently only around 4 per cent of babies are born on their due date and the later stages of pregnancy can feel like a waiting game as your baby's birth approaches. You may feel increasingly uncomfortable by this stage and getting to sleep is often difficult. As your baby gets ready to be born, they will usually start to move down into the pelvis ready for birth and you may experience Braxton Hicks contractions which are weak contractions of the womb as it gets ready for labour.

MULTIPLE BIRTHS

If you are expecting more than one baby, you will need additional care throughout your pregnancy as there is a higher risk of some complications for both you and your babies. You are likely to have more appointments and more scans. One of the main problems with a multiple pregnancy is that the babies are often born early, and your doctor or midwife will help you to weigh up whether you are likely to be able to give birth vaginally or should consider a Caesarean section. You will usually be advised that it would be best for you to give birth in a maternity unit in hospital just in case of any complications.

BREECH BABIES

Sometimes a baby does not move into position for birth but has its feet or bottom facing downwards as labour approaches. This is known as 'breech' and doctors may try to turn your baby by putting pressure on the womb. About half of all babies will turn using this method. You can also try using a technique from traditional Chinese medicine known as moxibustion (see Chapter 10, Complementary Therapies) to try to turn your baby, although the evidence on whether this works is limited. If your baby is still in a breech position, you will need to discuss the situation with the team caring for you to see whether you want to have a vaginal breech birth or to opt for a Caesarean section instead. This may depend on exactly how the baby is positioned and whether you have had any other pregnancy problems.

PROGRESS THROUGH LABOUR

The first sign of labour may be a 'show', when the mucus plug in the cervix that has protected the baby in pregnancy comes out and you may notice a pinky-red blob or blobs of discharge. This is not the same for everyone and you may feel contractions before anything else. For some women, the waters will break first. This happens when the amniotic sac breaks open and the fluid that surrounds the baby comes out through the vagina.

This time, before the contractions become very regular and strong, is known as the latent stage of labour and can last for many hours, or even longer in some cases. Once the contractions are closer together and longer, you are in the first stage of active labour and the cervix begins to open up (or dilate) more quickly. This stage of labour usually lasts up to five hours and is followed by transition, when the cervix gradually becomes fully dilated, contractions are very close together and much stronger and you get ready for the second stage of actively pushing the baby out. You will usually feel an urge to push as the baby moves down towards the vagina. This stage can last up to three hours if it is your first baby, but tends to be quite a bit quicker if you have given birth in the past. Sometimes women tear at this stage, or you may be given an episiotomy where a cut is made in the perineum (the area between the vagina and anus) to help the baby out, and you may need stitches afterwards.

After you have given birth to your baby, the placenta that has been nourishing the baby during pregnancy should follow shortly afterwards. You can have an injection to help the placenta to come out more quickly which will also reduce the risk of postpartum haemorrhage (very heavy bleeding after birth), but some women choose to try to wait for this to happen naturally.

In reality, giving birth doesn't always follow this neat pattern. Sometimes, particularly with first babies, things may be quite slow and if the team caring for you feels things are not progressing as they should, they may try to speed things up a little. They may offer to give you a vaginal examination and break your waters which can help if they haven't already broken. They can also give you

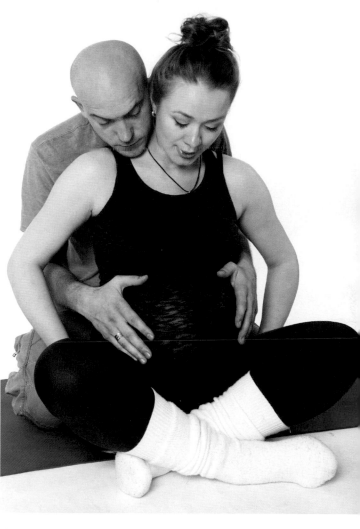

a drug (oxytocin or syntocinon) that makes the contractions stronger. It is given in a drip that goes into your arm or wrist and your baby will be monitored once this happens to make sure they are all right. Sometimes you may need a Caesarean section, even if you hadn't expected to have your baby this way.

CAESAREAN SECTION

If you know in advance you are going to have a Caesarean section it will be planned ahead so you know exactly when you are going to have your baby. Most often this will be for a medical reason, but some women choose to have their baby by Caesarean section. You will generally have a spinal anaesthetic so you can be awake throughout.

A cut is made across your belly just underneath your bikini line and your baby is usually born quickly and given to you to hold as soon as possible. Although it is a very common operation, a Caesarean section is major surgery and it will take you a while to get back to normal after the baby is born. You will probably need to stay in hospital for a little longer after a Caesarean section and you will need time to recover and painkillers. If you were expecting to have your baby vaginally but things don't go according to plan and there is a need to get the baby out quickly, you may need to have an emergency Caesarean section.

Sometimes women feel upset or disappointed if they have a Caesarean section when they had hoped to have a vaginal birth. If things had become quite frightening in the build-up to an emergency Caesarean or you have had to have a general anaesthetic this can leave you feeling quite traumatized. You may need some emotional support after the birth and if you are struggling, talk to your doctor, midwife or health visitor so they can make sure that you have the help you need.

STAYING HEALTHY IN THE RUN-UP TO GIVING BIRTH

You may find it a lot harder to get around in the last few weeks of pregnancy as by this stage you are likely to start to feel uncomfortable. It is great to still try to keep active unless your doctor has cautioned against this, but what you can do is likely to be limited by your size and what you feel comfortable with. Many women are still going for quite long walks or carrying on with yoga or swimming in the last month before they have their babies. Some are still at work until the very last few days before they have their babies. Even if you don't feel up to doing anything much in the final weeks of pregnancy, it is a good idea to get out every day if you can as this does help with your overall sense of wellbeing.

CHAPTER TWELVE

Beyond Birth: A Healthy Mother

When the Duchess of Cambridge appeared outside the hospital about seven hours after giving birth to Prince Louis looking glowing and glamorous, it gave a far from realistic vision of how most women look and feel shortly after having a baby. Giving birth is an exhausting and overwhelming experience and few would welcome the thought of having to be dressed immaculately and fully made-up for exposure to the world's media so soon afterwards. Many celebrity mothers seem to ping back to their pre-baby shape within days or weeks of having a baby, which can give the impression that this is somehow normal. Much more normal is to find that you look and feel exhausted and perhaps a bit stunned after giving birth. Although some women are elated and instantly bond with their baby, it doesn't always happen that way and you may feel traumatized if you have had a difficult birth. Your body will not just spring back to what it looked like before you had a baby but you will still have a bump, albeit a slightly smaller and saggier one, after the baby is born. You may have a tear, you may have stitches, you are likely to have bloody vaginal discharge, you may not be able to sit down and, if you have had a Caesarean section, you may not be able to move much at all for a while.

In the early days, your house is likely to be chaotic, your sleep patterns disrupted and you may spend days in your pyjamas with your hair unbrushed. A tiny baby looks so small and yet takes an impressive amount of time and effort to care for and many women find the first few days with their new baby a huge challenge as your life is turned upside down and you may find yourself swinging between elation and excitement and feeling full of anxiety and uncertainty about whether you are able to care for your newborn baby. This is all perfectly normal, and is most women's experience of the first days and weeks with a new baby.

Losing your baby weight and shape and getting back to the level of fitness you had before pregnancy is going to take time. If you are breastfeeding, you are likely to be hungrier than when you were pregnant as you need a lot more calories for your body to produce milk for your baby.

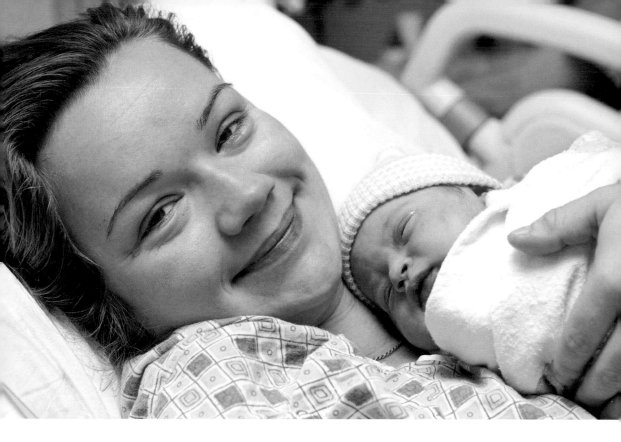

EMOTIONS AFTER GIVING BIRTH

We expect that we should feel happy when we have a newborn baby, but the huge hormonal changes that your body experiences after having a baby can lead to what is often known as the 'baby blues'. It may not feel right to be low when you have just had a baby but it may help to understand this is very normal and a majority of women will feel sad, irritable or tearful within a few days of giving birth. You have just been through an enormous physical and emotional experience and it can feel as if your entire lifestyle has been thrown up in the air with the arrival of your baby. If you add to that post-birth pain and discomfort, feeling exhausted and foggy-brained due to lack of sleep and uncertainty as to whether you are tending to your newborn baby's needs as you should be, it is hardly surprising that the joy of having your baby can get drowned out by some of the other emotions you are experiencing.

To some extent, these confused feelings in the early days after birth are inevitable, but there are some things you can do to make a difference:

- Try not to be hard on yourself or to have unrealistic expectations about what you should be achieving and how you are feeling. Not being able to find time to do the washing, or even the washing-up, is perfectly normal. If you are someone who likes to have a spotless house it may not be easy to let go, but things will get easier with time as you adjust to life with your baby.

- Make sure you get as much rest as you can. If your baby is having an afternoon nap, you should try to have one too rather than trying to fit in a few domestic tasks while your baby sleeps.
- Do not feel that you need to be immaculately dressed and getting out and about within days of your baby's birth but allow yourself time to recover; listen to your own body.
- Make sure you are eating properly. It is surprisingly easy to forget to eat when your normal daytime routines are dominated by your baby but it is just as important to eat properly now, especially if you are breastfeeding. This is not the time to start any kind of post-pregnancy diet either, as your body needs to recover and you need all the energy you can get. Sometimes if your schedule is all over the place it can be tempting to fill up on biscuits or other quick snacks rather than eating proper meals, but try to eat a balanced diet with plenty of fresh vegetables and fruit.
- Accept offers of help! If you have relatives or friends around who are asking if they can do anything, why not ask them to load the dishwasher or make you a cup of tea? If family and friends are keen to give you a hand in the early days it can make all the difference, and don't forget that people like to feel needed.
- You should never feel pressured to get out and about until you are ready, but once you are up to it, getting outside for just a short walk and some fresh air can be really beneficial.

POSTNATAL DEPRESSION

The phase of feeling low after having your baby, known as the baby blues, usually lasts for about ten to fourteen days. If you continue to be depressed after this and things do not seem to be improving with time, talk to someone about how you are feeling. This may be your partner or a friend first, but there are some signs that you may be experiencing postnatal depression and if you feel these describe how you are feeling beyond the first few weeks, you should get medical help.

These signs may include the following:

- You are tearful and cry a lot
- You are constantly irritable and tense
- You feel you can no longer enjoy anything in life
- You find it hard to get to sleep
- You are exhausted and do not have any energy
- Your appetite is affected and you are comfort-eating or have a poor appetite
- You find it hard to cope and are feeling overwhelmed
- You feel isolated and lonely
- You are unable to concentrate and find it hard to make decisions

- You are constantly blaming yourself for not being a good enough mother and are having difficulty bonding with your baby
- You have experienced panic attacks.

Not everyone will experience all of these, but if this feels familiar to you, then getting help is really important. It can be difficult to talk to a doctor or health visitor about all this, but if you do they can help and you may be be offered some kind of support to help you to feel better.

BREASTFEEDING

We know breastfeeding has many benefits for your baby as breast milk contains everything they need and can help to protect them against some common ailments such as colds and diarrhoea. It can have long-term health benefits for your baby, reducing the chances of childhood leukemia, of obesity later in life and of cardiovascular disease, and for you too, cutting your chances of breast and ovarian cancer, osteoporosis, cardiovascular disease and obesity. Apart from that, breast milk is free and always there for your baby when they need or want it.

For many women, breastfeeding is not as easy as they were expecting and sore or cracked nipples and pain when feeding can make it a far from enjoyable experience in the early days. There is support for breastfeeding and it is really worth giving it a go and getting help if you need it. Difficulties feeding can be down to getting your baby into the right position, and to you and your baby getting used to breastfeeding. It does get easier with time and perseverance can pay off. This doesn't always happen

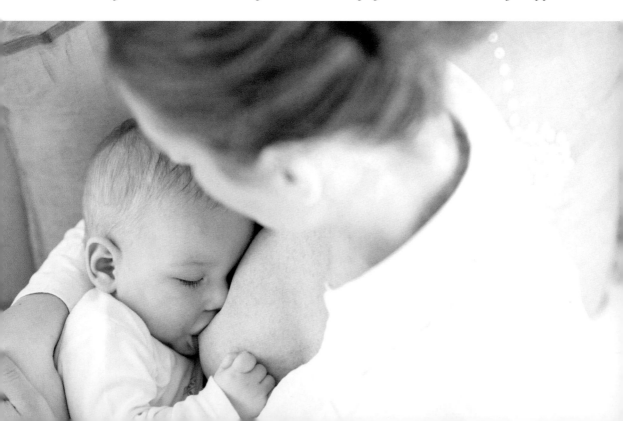

though and some women struggle to feed despite having advice and support. If it continues to be painful and is causing both you and your baby distress or if your baby is becoming dehydrated, you may need to offer formula instead.

If this is your experience, you should not feel guilty or blame yourself as it does sometimes happen. There may be medical reasons why you can't breastfeed, for example if you are HIV positive or are taking certain types of medication. Other people can sometimes be judgemental about bottle-feeding and formula, but quite frankly it has nothing to do with them. Formula is not going to harm your baby and the decision to bottle-feed is yours alone.

BUILDING UP TO EXERCISE

It is very easy to be focused on your baby in the weeks after birth and to almost forget about yourself, but looking after you is essential if you are to be able to look after your baby. It is likely to take a few weeks before you are feeling anything like normal again, but you can start being more active when you feel ready for this after the birth.

You will continue bleeding after giving birth and the discharge, known as lochia, will gradually get paler in the weeks following the birth. If you are too active too quickly, you can make this bleeding heavier so it is important to start gently and gradually build up your levels of exercise rather than pushing yourself to over-achieve from the start.

The one thing you really should start doing sooner rather than later is pelvic floor exercises as it is important to start strengthening your pelvic floor muscles. Even with these, you need to start gradually as they can be uncomfortable if you have had a tear, stitches or an episiotomy. After giving birth, you may experience some stress incontinence when you leak urine if you sneeze or cough or take physical exercise, and pelvic floor exercises can help with this.

Exercise after a Caesarean Section

If you have had a Caesarean section, you will be given advice from the hospital about what you can do after the operation and when. Initially it is likely to feel very uncomfortable and you may not be able to do much at all. As you gradually recover, you should allow yourself time rather than pushing yourself to do more too quickly. The recovery period is normally estimated at around six weeks, and you should be particularly careful to avoid any heavy lifting. Once you start to feel a bit better, walking is a great first exercise but you need to allow yourself time to start slowly and build up your strength and flexibility.

A FIT AND HEALTHY MOTHER

The first exercise you will want to take after giving birth is simply walking. It is the ideal post-birth exercise and you can start slowly with short distances and gradually build up. What's even better is the fact that you can take your baby with you, either in a pram or a sling. It is often recommended you wait until after your six-week check (or eight-week check for a Caesarean) before doing any more strenuous exercise. Although very fit athletes may feel ready to get back to exercise before this, if you are a recreational exerciser or someone who hadn't been that active before you became pregnant, take your time and only do what feels right. If there have been complications during the pregnancy and/or birth, always take medical advice about how soon you can start exercising and what you should do.

If you are lucky, you may find some local mother-and-baby exercise classes you can go to such as yoga or Pilates. There are more and more of these classes available now, but accessing them can depend on where you live and there may be more options if you are in a town or city. You may also want to consider mother-and-baby swimming classes once your baby has had all their vaccinations. Swimming is a good gentle exercise for you to start with too, but you need to wait until you have stopped bleeding and any scars from a Caesarean section or an episiotomy, or any tears, are healed. Some local leisure centres run special postnatal aqua fitness classes and these may be a good way of getting back into being active.

With high-impact exercise like running, you need to be more cautious and you may want to start with power-walking and then gradually include short phases of slow jogging as you build up your confidence and strength. When you can start running again is very much dependent on how you are recovering from giving birth and also how fit you were beforehand. The general advice from pelvic health physiotherapists is that you should wait at least twelve weeks before doing running or star jumps.

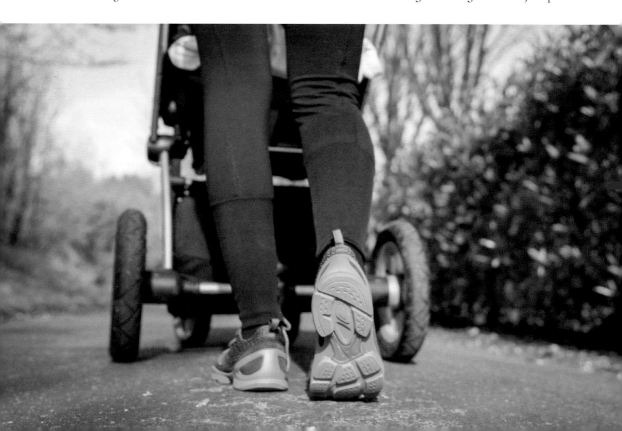

If you have had any leaking or continence problems, if you have pelvic or lower back pain or if you have any bulging or straining from your abdomen or vagina, you should be more cautious as these signs suggest you may not be ready to run. If you have any concerns, always talk to your doctor or health visitor before you start running again and always ease yourself back gently, stopping if you experience any discomfort or bleeding. It is also vital to make sure you are wearing a comfortable and well-fitted bra while you are still breastfeeding and to make sure you drink plenty of water as it is easy to get dehydrated when you are feeding your baby.

The same guidance goes for getting back into the gym and any exercise classes. The key thing is to ease yourself back in gradually. Don't expect too much of yourself at first, and don't feel embarrassed to be the person at the back of the class who leaves out anything too challenging; it is all about following what your body is telling you. The important thing is not to try to push yourself hard into too much exercise as your body needs time to rest and recover after carrying a baby for nine months and giving birth.

One of the things that may be difficult when you have a new baby is simply finding the time to exercise, and that's why walking or running which you can do with a baby in a buggy can be particularly appealing. Alternatively, your local gym or fitness centre may have a crèche where you can leave your baby for an hour while you go to a class or have a workout. If you are finding it really hard to get out and about, you may want to ask a family member or friend to do an hour's babysitting for you as being active after your baby's birth will not only improve your physical health, it will help to give you energy and can benefit your mental health, reducing anxiety. It can improve your overall sense of wellbeing to get out and about and to do something for yourself.

Although taking some time out for you to keep fit and active when you have a small baby may feel self-centred, the benefits of this are not just for you. Having a happier and healthier mother is good for your whole family, and if your children grow up seeing the value of a healthy lifestyle, the health benefits of eating well and keeping active will pass on to the next generation.

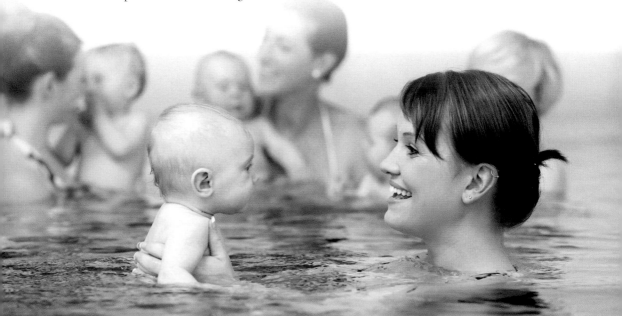

Index

exercise 7-10, 27, 40-55, 57-61, 72, 77, 80-82, 85, 87-88, 99-100, 111-13

exhaustion 9, 42-43, 47, 56, 86, 107-9